Oncologic Ultrasound

Editor

VIKRAM DOGRA

ULTRASOUND CLINICS

www.ultrasound.theclinics.com

Consulting Editor
VIKRAM DOGRA

January 2014 • Volume 9 • Number 1

ELSEVIER

1600 John F. Kennedy Boulevard • Suite 1800 • Philadelphia, Pennsylvania, 19103-2899

http://www.theclinics.com

ULTRASOUND CLINICS Volume 9, Number 1
January 2014 ISSN 1556-858X, ISBN-13: 978-0-323-26416-7

Editor: John Vassallo
Developmental Editor: Stephanie Carter

Ultrasound Clinics (ISSN 1556-858X) is published quarterly by Elsevier, Inc., 360 Park Avenue South, New York, NY 10010-1710. Months of publication are January, April, July, and October. Business and editorial offices: 1600 John F. Kennedy Boulevard, Suite 1800, Philadelphia, Pennsylvania 19103-2899. Accounting and circulation offices: 6277 Sea Harbor Drive, Orlando, FL 32887-4800. Periodicals postage paid at New York, NY, and additional mailing offices. Subscription prices are $270 per year for (US individuals), $327 per year for (US institutions), $130 per year for (US students and residents), $305 per year for (Canadian individuals), $369 per year for (Canadian institutions), $325 per year for (international individuals), $369 per year for (international institutions), and $155 per year for (Canadian and foreign students/residents). To receive student/resident rate, orders must be accompanied by name of affiliated institution, date of term, and the signature of program/residency coordinator on institution letterhead. Orders will be billed at individual rate until proof of status is received. Foreign air speed delivery is included in all Clinics subscription prices. All prices are subject to change without notice. **POSTMASTER:** Send address changes to *Ultrasound Clinics,* Elsevier Health Sciences Division, Subscription Customer Service, 3251 Riverport Lane, Maryland Heights, MO 63043. **Customer Service (orders, claims, online, change of address): Telephone: 1-800-654-2452 (U.S. and Canada); 314-447-8871 (outside U.S. and Canada). Fax: 314-447-8029. E-mail: journalscustomerservice-usa@elsevier.com (for print support); journalsonlinesupport-usa@elsevier.com (for online support).**

Reprints: For copies of 100 or more, of articles in this publication, please contact the Commercial Reprints Department, Elsevier Inc., 360 Park Avenue South, New York, NY 10010-1710. Tel.: (+1) 212-633-3874; Fax: (+1) 212-633-3820; E-mail: reprints@elsevier.com.

Printed and bound by CPI Group (UK) Ltd, Croydon, CR0 4YY

Transferred to digital print 2013

Contributors

CONSULTING EDITOR

VIKRAM DOGRA, MD
Professor of Radiology, Urology, and
Biomedical Engineering, Associate Chair
for Education and Research, Director of
Ultrasound, Department of Imaging Sciences,
University of Rochester School of Medicine,
Rochester, New York

EDITOR

VIKRAM DOGRA, MD
Professor of Radiology, Urology and
Biomedical Engineering, Associate Chair of
Education and Research, Director of
Ultrasound, Department of Imaging Sciences,
University of Rochester School of Medicine,
Rochester, New York

AUTHORS

MARCO A. ALVAREZ, MD
Diagnostic Radiology and Imaging, Alvarez
and Arrazola Radiólogos, Mazatlán, Sinaloa,
México

DEVANG BUTANI, MD
Assistant Professor, Division of Interventional
Radiology, Department of Imaging Sciences,
University of Rochester Medical Center,
Rochester, New York

MANJIRI K. DIGHE, MD
Associate Professor, Department of Radiology,
University of Washington, Seattle, Washington

VIKRAM DOGRA, MD
Professor of Radiology, Urology and
Biomedical Engineering, Associate Chair
of Education and Research, Director of
Ultrasound, Department of Imaging Sciences,
University of Rochester School of Medicine,
Rochester, New York

MARVIN M. DOYLEY, PhD
Department of Electrical and Computer
Engineering, University of Rochester,
Rochester, New York

DAVID C. HOWLETT, FRCP, FRCR
Consultant Radiologist, Honorary Reader,
Brighton and Sussex Medical School,
Honorary Senior Lecturer, Kings College
London, East Sussex Hospitals NHS Trust,
Eastbourne District General Hospital,
Radiology Department, Eastbourne, East
Sussex, United Kingdom

VIVEK KAUL, MD, FACG
Associate Professor of Medicine,
Chief, Division of Gastroenterology
and Hepatology, Center for Advanced
Therapeutic Endoscopy, University
of Rochester Medical Center/Strong
Memorial Hospital, Rochester, New York

SHIVANGI KOTHARI, MD
Assistant Professor of Medicine, Division
of Gastroenterology and Hepatology,
Associate Director of Endoscopy, Center for
Advanced Therapeutic Endoscopy, University
of Rochester Medical Center/Strong Memorial
Hospital, Rochester, New York

**UDAY Y. MANDALIA, MBBS, BSc,
MRCPCH, FRCR**
Radiology Registrar, Radiology Department,
Guys and St Thomas' NHS Trust, St Thomas'
Hospital, London, United Kingdom

MEHMET RUHI ONUR, MD
Associate Professor of Radiology, Department
of Radiology, School of Medicine, University
of Firat, Elazig, Turkey

KEVIN J. PARKER, PhD
Department of Electrical and Computer
Engineering, University of Rochester,
Rochester, New York

FRANCOIS N. PORTE, MBBS, FRCR
Radiology Registrar, Radiology
Department, Guys and St Thomas'
NHS Trust, St Thomas' Hospital, London,
United Kingdom

JOSEPH REIS, MD
Fellow, Division of Interventional Radiology,
Department of Imaging Sciences, University
of Rochester Medical Center, Rochester,
New York

AHMET TUNCAY TURGUT, MD
Associate Professor of Radiology,
Department of Radiology, Ankara Training
and Research Hospital, Ankara, Turkey

STEPHANIE R. WILSON, MD
Clinical Professor of Radiology, Clinical
Professor of Gastroenterology, University
of Calgary, Alberta, Canada

Contents

Endoscopic ultrasound (EUS) has evolved from a purely diagnostic modality to one with potential for multiple therapeutic applications. These interventional EUS techniques are minimally invasive and have emerged as a safe alternative to radiologic and surgical approaches. Techniques such as celiac plexus neurolysis for analgesia, EUS-guided endoscopic retrograde cholangiopancreatography for difficult-to-access bile ducts obstructed by tumor or due to difficult anatomy, EUS guided fiducial placement to help guide radiation therapy, and delivery of antitumor agents are just some of the therapeutic applications of EUS in patients with cancer. In this article, the various EUS-guided therapeutic interventions currently used in clinical practice and other investigational interventions in the realm of pancreatic neoplasia management are discussed.

Ablation is a minimally invasive procedure used to treat both cancerous and noncancerous conditions. Contrast-enhanced ultrasonography and sonoelastography have significantly improved lesion visualization before, during, and after ablation. The use of various imaging modalities and ablative techniques is encouraged to allow appropriate individualization of treatment. This review focuses on ultrasonographic applications for 2 common methods of ablation, namely radiofrequency ablation and cryoablation, in treating hepatic and renal tumors. Brief mention is made of microwave ablation and irreversible electroporation.

The main indications for transrectal ultrasound (TRUS)-guided prostate biopsy are abnormal digital rectal examination or increased prostate-specific antigen level. TRUS-guided prostate biopsy involves sampling 12 cores from midparasagittal and lateral aspects of the base, midgland, and apex of the prostate. Saturation biopsy should be reserved for repeat biopsy in the setting of negative results on initial biopsy in patients who are still strongly suspected to have prostate cancer. Advanced imaging techniques can be used in targeted prostate biopsy to increase sensitivity of biopsy in the detection of cancer and decrease the number of biopsy cores.

Prostate cancer is among the top newly diagnosed cancers. Its approach has radically shifted because of the prostate-specific antigen, transrectal ultrasound-guided biopsy (TRUS), and improvements in medical and surgical options. The use of biomarkers for prostate cancer screening helps not only to select which patients will likely benefit from TRUS but also to discriminate between aggressive and indolent disease once the diagnosis is confirmed.

As superficial structures, the salivary glands are easily assessed by ultrasound. This article reviews the role of imaging in the management of salivary gland tumors, with an emphasis on the use of ultrasound. The anatomy of the major salivary glands, the technique of salivary gland ultrasound, and the typical appearances of the common benign and malignant lesions are discussed. In addition, the use of ultrasound-guided interventional techniques and ultrasound elastography of salivary gland tumors is discussed.

ULTRASOUND CLINICS

RELATED INTEREST

November 2012, Volume 50, Issue 6
Radiologic Clinics of North America
Imaging of Lung Cancer
Baskaran Sundaram, MBBS, MRCP, FRCR, and Ella A. Kazerooni, MD, MS, FACR, *Editors*

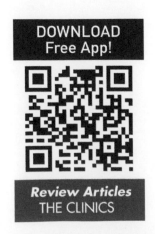

DOWNLOAD
Free App!

Review Articles
THE CLINICS

NOW AVAILABLE FOR YOUR iPhone and iPad

PROGRAM OBJECTIVE

The goal of the *Ultrasound Clinics* is to keep practicing radiologists and radiology residents up to date with current clinical practice in ultrasound by providing timely articles reviewing the state of the art in patient care.

TARGET AUDIENCE

Practicing radiologists, radiology residents and other healthcare professionals who provide care based on radiologic findings.

LEARNING OBJECTIVES

Upon completion of this activity, participants will be able to:
1. Describe ultrasound guidance in tumor ablation.
2. Review the general principles and clinical applications of elastography.
3. Discuss endoscopic ultrasound in oncology.

ACCREDITATION

The Elsevier Office of Continuing Medical Education (EOCME) is accredited by the Accreditation Council for Continuing Medical Education (ACCME) to provide continuing medical education for physicians.

The EOCME designates this enduringmaterial for a maximum of 15 *AMA PRA Category 1 Credit*(s)™. Physicians should claim only the credit commensurate with the extent of their participation in the activity.

All other health care professionals requesting continuing education credit for this enduring material will be issued a certificate of participation.

DISCLOSURE OF CONFLICTS OF INTEREST

The EOCME assesses conflict of interest with its instructors, faculty, planners, and other individuals who are in a position to control the content of CME activities. All relevant conflicts of interest that are identified are thoroughly vetted by EOCME for fair balance, scientific objectivity, and patient care recommendations. EOCME is committed to providing its learners with CME activities that promote improvements or quality in healthcare and not a specific proprietary business or a commercial interest.

The planning committee, staff, authors and editors listed below have identified no financial relationships or relationships to products or devices they or their spouse/life partner have with commercial interest related to the content of this CME activity:

Marco A. Alvarez, MD; Devang Butani, MD; Stephanie Carter; Joseph Daniel; Vikram Dogra, MD; Marvin M. Doyley, PhD; Kristen Helm; David C. Howlett, FRCP, FRCR; Brynne Hunter; Shivangi Kothari, MD; Vivek Kaul, MD, FACG; Sandy Lavery; Uday Y. Mandalia MBBS, BSc, MRCPCH, FRCR; Jill McNair; Mehmet Ruhi Onur, MD; Kevin J. Parker, PhD; Francois N. Porte, MBBS, FRCR; Joseph Reis, MD; Ahmet Tuncay Turgut, MD; John Vassallo.

The planning committee, staff, authors and editors listed below have identified financial relationships or relationships to products or devices they or their spouse/life partner have with commercial interest related to the content of this CME activity:

Manjiri K. Dighe, MD is conducting a NIH R21 study on Shear wave elastography in thyroid nodules.

Stephanie R. Wilson, MD is consultant/advisor for Lantheus Medical Imaging; has research grants from Lantheus Medical Imaging, AbbViePharma, and Janssen Pharmaceuticals Inc.

UNAPPROVED/OFF-LABEL USE DISCLOSURE

The EOCME requires CME faculty to disclose to the participants:
1. When products or procedures being discussed are off-label, unlabelled, experimental, and/or investigational (not US Food and Drug Administration (FDA) approved); and
2. Any limitations on the information presented, such as data that are preliminary or that represent ongoing research, interim analyses, and/or unsupported opinions. Faculty may discuss information about pharmaceutical agents that is outside of FDA-approved labelling. This information is intended solely for CME and is not intended to promote off-label use of these medications. If you have any questions, contact the medical affairs department of the manufacturer for the most recent prescribing information.

TO ENROLL

To enroll in the *Ultrasounds Clinic* Continuing Medical Education program, call customer service at 1-800-654-2452 or sign up online at http://www.theclinics.com/home/cme. The CME program is available to subscribers for an additional annual fee of USD 212.

METHOD OF PARTICIPATION

In order to claim credit, participants must complete the following:
1. Complete enrolment as indicated above.
2. Read the activity.
3. Complete the CME Test and Evaluation. Participants must achieve a score of 70% on the test. All CME Tests and Evaluations must be completed online.

CME INQUIRIES/SPECIAL NEEDS

For all CME inquiries or special needs, please contact elsevierCME@elsevier.com.

Preface

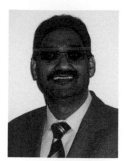

Vikram Dogra, MD
Editor

It is my pleasure to introduce this new issue of *Ultrasound Clinics* dedicated to oncology. Ultrasound is widely used in oncologic imaging because of its nonradiation properties. There have been new developments in oncologic imaging such as elastography, and an introductory article on elastography has been included in this issue, including its applications in thyroid disease.

This issue of *Ultrasound Clinics* covers the latest developments in endoscopic ultrasound and its therapeutic applications. A special article has been included on new biomarkers of prostate cancer. Other topics of interest in this issue are salivary gland imaging, ultrasound-guided prostate biopsy, and ultrasound guidance in tumor ablation.

I want to thank our contributors for their outstanding work.

With best wishes,

Vikram Dogra, MD
University of Rochester School of Medicine
Department of Imaging Sciences
601 Elmwood Avenue, Box 648
Rochester, NY 14642, USA

E-mail address:
Vikram_Dogra@URMC.Rochester.edu

Ultrasound Clin 9 (2014) xi
http://dx.doi.org/10.1016/j.cult.2013.09.003
1556-858X/14/$ – see front matter © 2014 Elsevier Inc. All rights reserved.

Elastography
General Principles and Clinical Applications

Marvin M. Doyley, PhD*, Kevin J. Parker, PhD

KEYWORDS

- Elastography • Ultrasonic imaging • Ultrasonic elastography • MRI

KEY POINTS

- Like conventional medical imaging modalities, forward and the inverse problems are encountered in elastography.
- Quasistatic elastography visualizes the strain induced within tissue using either an external or internal source.
- Direct and iterative inversion schemes have been developed to make quasistatic elastograms more quantitative.
- Soft tissues display several biomechanical properties, including viscosity and nonlinearity, which may improve the diagnostic value of elastography when visualized alone or in combination with shear modulus. Elastography can characterize the nonlinear behavior of soft tissues and may be used to differentiate between benign and malignant tumors.

INTRODUCTION

Elastography visualizes differences in the biomechanical properties of normal and diseased tissues.[1–4] Elastography was developed in the late 1980s to early 1990s to improve ultrasonic imaging,[5–7] but the success of ultrasonic elastography has inspired investigators to develop analogs based on MRI[8–11] and optical coherence tomography.[12–14] This article focuses on ultrasonic techniques with a brief reference to approaches based on MRI.

The general principles of elastography can be summarized as follows: (1) perturb the tissue using a quasistatic, harmonic, or transient mechanical source; (2) measure the resulting mechanical response (displacement, strain or amplitude, and phase of vibration); and (3) infer the biomechanical properties of the underlying tissue by applying either a simplified or continuum mechanical model to the measured mechanical response.[2,15–18] This article describes (1) the general principles of quasistatic, harmonic, and transient elastography

(Fig. 1)—the most popular approaches to elastography—and (2) the physics of elastography—the underlying equations of motion that govern the motion in each approach. Examples of clinical applications of each approach are provided.

THE PHYSICS OF ELASTOGRAPHY

Like conventional medical imaging modalities, forward and the inverse problems are encountered in elastography. The former problems are concerned with predicting the mechanical response of a material with known biomechanical properties and external boundary conditions. Understanding these problems and devising accurate theoretical models to solve them have been an effective strategy in developing and optimizing the performance of ultrasound displacement estimation methods. The latter problems are concerned with estimating biomechanical properties noninvasively using the forward model and knowledge of the mechanical response and external boundary conditions. A comprehensive review of methods developed to

Department of Electrical and Computer Engineering, University of Rochester, Hopeman Engineering Building 343, Box 270126, Rochester, NY 14627, USA
* Corresponding author.
E-mail address: m.doyley@rochester.edu

Ultrasound Clin 9 (2014) 1–11
http://dx.doi.org/10.1016/j.cult.2013.09.006
1556-858X/14/$ – see front matter Published by Elsevier Inc.

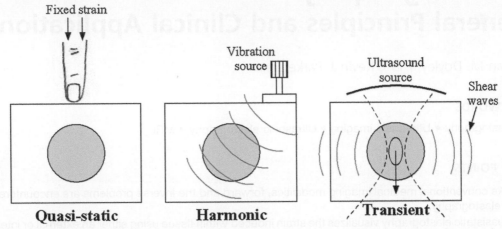

Fig. 1. Schematic representation of current approaches to elastographic imaging: quasistatic elastography (*left*), harmonic elastography (*middle*), and transient elastography (*right*).

solve inverse problems is given in the article by Doyley[19]; therefore, this section focuses only on the forward problem.

The forward elastography problem can be described by a system of partial differential equations (PDEs) given in compact form[20,21]:

$$\nabla \times \left[\sigma_{ij}\right] = \beta_i \tag{1}$$

where σ_{ij} is the 3-D stress tensor (ie, a vector of vectors), β_i is the deforming force, and ∇ is the del operator. Using the assumption that soft tissues exhibit linear elastic behavior, then the strain tensor (ε) maybe related to the stress tensor (σ) as follows[22]:

$$\sigma_{ij} = C_{ijkl}\varepsilon_{kl} \tag{2}$$

where the tensor (C) is a rank-four tensor consisting of 21 independent elastic constants.[16,20,23] Under the assumption that soft tissues exhibit isotropic mechanical behavior, however, then only 2 independent constants, λ and μ (lambda and shear modulus), are required. The relationship between stress and strain for linear isotropic elastic materials is given by:

$$\sigma_{ij} = 2\mu\varepsilon_{ij} + \lambda\delta_{ij}\Theta \tag{3}$$

where $\Theta = \nabla \cdot \mathbf{u} = \varepsilon_{11} + \varepsilon_{22} + \varepsilon_{33}$ is the compressibility relation, δ is the Kronecker delta, and the components of the strain tensor are defined as:

$$\varepsilon_{ij} = \frac{1}{2}\left(\frac{\partial u_i}{\partial j} + \frac{\partial u_j}{\partial x_i}\right) \tag{4}$$

Lamé constants (ie, λ and μ) are related to Young modulus (E) and Poisson ratio (v), as follows[20,21]:

$$\mu = \frac{E}{2(1+v)}, \quad \lambda = \frac{vE}{(1+v)(1-2v)} \tag{5}$$

The stress tensor is eliminated from the equilibrium equations (ie, Equation 2) using Equation 3. The strain components are then expressed in terms of displacements using Equation 4. The resulting equations (ie, the Navier-Stokes equations) are given by:

$$\nabla \cdot \mu\nabla\mathbf{u} + \nabla(\lambda+\mu)\nabla \cdot \mathbf{u} = \rho\frac{\partial^2 \mathbf{u}}{\partial t^2} \tag{6}$$

where ρ the is density of the material, $\mathbf{u}$ is the displacement vector, and t is time. For quasistatic deformations, Equation 6 reduces to:

$$\nabla \cdot \mu\nabla\mathbf{u} + \nabla(\lambda+\mu)\nabla \cdot \mathbf{u} = 0 \tag{7}$$

For harmonic deformations, the time-independent (steady-state) equations in the frequency domain give[10,24]:

$$\nabla \cdot \mu\nabla\mathbf{u} + \nabla(\lambda+\mu)\nabla \cdot \mathbf{u} = \rho\omega^2\mathbf{u} \tag{8}$$

where ω is the angular frequency of the sinusoidal excitation. For transient deformations, the wave equation is derived by differentiating Equation 6 with respect to x, y, and z, which gives[21]:

$$\nabla^2\Delta = \frac{1}{c_1^2}\frac{\partial^2\Delta}{\partial t^2} \tag{9}$$

where $\nabla \cdot \mathbf{u} = \Delta$, and the velocity of the propagating compressional wave, c_1, is given by:

$$c_1 = \sqrt{\frac{\lambda+2\mu}{\rho}} \tag{10}$$

The wave equation for the propagating shear wave is given by:

$$\nabla^2\zeta = \frac{1}{c_2^2}\frac{\partial^2\zeta}{\partial t^2} \tag{11}$$

where $\zeta = \nabla \cdot u/2$ is the rotational vector, and the shear wave velocity, c_2, is given by:

$$c_2 = \sqrt{\frac{\mu}{\rho}} \qquad (12)$$

Analytical methods have been used to solve the governing equations for quasistatic, harmonic, and transient elastographic imaging methods[25–28] for simple geometries and boundary conditions. Numeric methods—namely, the finite-element method—are used, however, to solve the governing equations for all 3 approaches to elastography on irregular domains and for heterogeneous elasticity distributions.[24,29–36]

APPROACHES TO ELASTOGRAPHY
Quasistatic Elastography

Quasistatic elastography visualizes the strain induced within tissue using either an external or internal source. A small motion is induced within the tissue (typically approximately 2% of the axial dimension) with a quasistatic mechanical source. The axial component of the internal tissue displacement is measured by performing cross-correlation analysis on pre- and postdeformed radiofrequency (RF) echo frames[6,7,37] and strain is estimated by spatially differentiating the axial displacements. In quasistatic elastography, soft tissues are typically viewed as a series of 1-D springs that are arranged in a simple fashion. For this simple mechanical model, the measured strain (ε) is related to the internal stress (σ) by Hooke's law:

$$\sigma = k\varepsilon \qquad (13)$$

where k is the Young modulus (or stiffness) of the tissue. No method can measure the internal stress distribution in vivo; consequently, the internal stress distribution is assumed to be constant (ie, $\sigma \approx 1$); an approximate estimate of Young modulus is computed from the reciprocal of the measured strain. The disadvantage of computing modulus elastograms in this manner is that it does not account for stress decay or stress concentration; consequently, quasistatic elastograms typically contain target-hardening artifacts,[31,35] as illustrated in **Fig. 2**.

Despite this limitation, several groups have obtained good elastograms in applications where accurate quantification of Young modulus is not essential. For example, **Fig. 3** shows the results of a case study, where quasistatic elastography was performed on a 73-year-old woman with a phyllodes tumor in the upper outer quadrant of her left breast. Phyllodes tumors are rare variants of fibroadenoma, with a rich stromal component and more cellularity. They grow quickly, developing macroscopically lobulated internal structures and may reach a large size, visibly altering the breast profile. Sonography generally shows a solid, moderately hypoechoic nodule with smooth borders and good sound transmission.[38] Inhomogenous structures may be present because of small internal fluid areas. These appearances are nonspecific, and sonography is not currently able to distinguish between benign and malignant cases, nor can it make a differential diagnosis between fibroadenoma and phyllodes tumors.

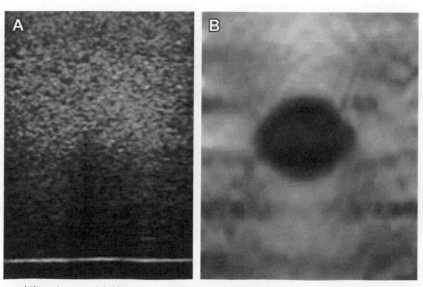

Fig. 2. Sonogram (*A*) and strain (*B*) elastograms obtained from a phantom containing a single 10-mm diameter inclusion whose modulus contrast was approximately 6.03 dB.

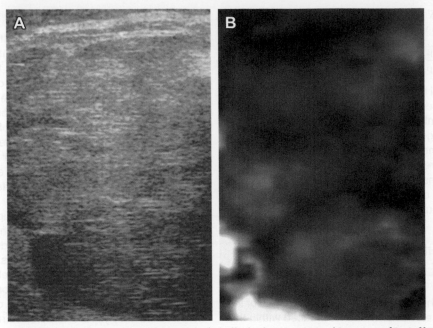

Fig. 3. Sonographic (*A*) and elastographic (*B*) images of phyllodes breast tumor. (*Courtesy of* Dr Jeff Bamber, Institute of Cancer Research in London, London, England.)

In the sonogram shown in **Fig. 3**, the tumor covers most of the field of view, with the capsule of the anterior margin visible close to the top of the image and the posterior margin visible at the bottom left. Within the tumor, the appearance is heterogeneous on a large scale, with macroscopic lobules separated by echogenic boundaries that are probably fibrous in nature. The strain elastogram (see **Fig. 3**B) confirms this appearance but shows it much more clearly with greater contrast than the sonogram (see **Fig. 3**A). The macroscopic lobules within the tumor are clearly defined as soft regions separated by stiff septa, which is consistent with the septa being of a fibrous nature.

Direct and iterative inversion schemes have been developed to make quasistatic elastograms more quantitative. These techniques compute

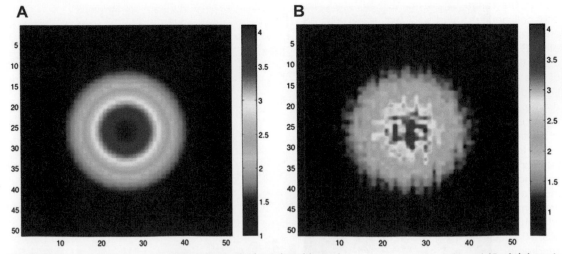

Fig. 4. Modulus elastograms computed from ideal axial and lateral strain estimates (*A, left*) and (*B, right*) strain estimates that were corrupted with 4% additive white noise. The simulated phantom contained an inclusion with a gaussian modulus distribution that had a peak contrast of 4:1. (*Courtesy of* Dr P. Barbone, Boston University Department of Mechanical and Aeronautic Engineering, Boston, MA.)

the Young's or shear modulus from the measured displacement or strain using the forward elasticity model described in Equation 7. Direct inversion schemes use a linear system of equations derived by rearranging the PDEs that describe the forward elastography problem.[8,28,39]

$$(\partial_{yy} - \partial_{xx})(\varepsilon_{xy}\mu) + \partial_{xy}(\varepsilon_{xy}\mu) = 0 \tag{14}$$

Equation 14 contains high-order derivatives that amplify measurement noise, which compromises the quality of ensuing modulus elastograms, as demonstrated in **Fig. 4**.

Iterative inversion techniques[40,41] overcome this issue by considering the inverse problem as a parameter-optimization task, where the goal is to find the Young's modulus that minimizes the error between measured displacement or strain fields and those computed by solving the forward elastography problem. The matrix solution at the $(k + 1)$ iteration that has the general form:

$$\mu^{k+1} = \Delta\mu^k + \left[J(\mu^k)^T J(\mu^k) + \rho I\right]^{-1} J(\mu^k)^T (u_m - u\{\mu^k\}) \tag{15}$$

where $\Delta\mu^k$ is a vector of shear modulus updates at all coordinates in the reconstruction field and J is the Jacobian, or sensitivity, matrix. The Hessian matrix, $[J(\mu^k)^T J(\mu^k)]$, is ill conditioned. Therefore, to stabilize performance in the presence of measurement noise, the matrix is regularized using 1 of 3 variational methods: the Tikhonov,[41] the Marquardt,[42] or the total variational method.[43,44] **Fig. 5** shows an example of modulus elastograms computed with the iterative inversion approach.

The contrast-to-noise ratio of the modulus elastogram is better than that of the strain elastogram, which improved the detection of the boundary between the ablated region and normal tissue to enable accurate determination of the size of the thermal zone.

Harmonic Elastography Based on Local Frequency Estimation

In harmonic elastography,[5,5–9,34,45] low-frequency acoustic waves (typically <1 kHz) are transmitted within the tissue using a sinusoidal mechanical source. The phase and amplitude of the propagating waves are visualized using either color Doppler imaging[34,45,46] (**Fig. 6**) or phase-contrast MRI.[9–11]

Assuming that shear waves propagate with plane wave fronts, then an approximate estimate of the local shear modulus (μ) may be computed from local estimates of the wavelength:

$$v_{shear} = \sqrt{\frac{\mu}{\rho}} \tag{16}$$

where v_{shear} is the velocity of the shear wave, and ρ is the density of the tissue. In a homogeneous tissue, shear modulus can be estimated from local estimates of instantaneous frequency.[47,48] Although shear modulus estimated using this approach is insensitive to measurement noise, the spatial resolution of the ensuing modulus elastograms is limited. A further weakness of the approach is that the plane wave approximation breaks down in complex organs, such as the breast and brain, when waves reflected from internal tissue boundaries interfere constructively and destructively.

Like quasistatic elastography, solving the inverse elastography problem improves the performance of harmonic elastography. **Fig. 7** shows a representative example of an elastogram obtained from a healthy volunteer by solving the inverse harmonic elastography problem. The resolution of the elastograms was sufficiently high to visualize fibroglandular tissue from the adipose tissue.[49,50]

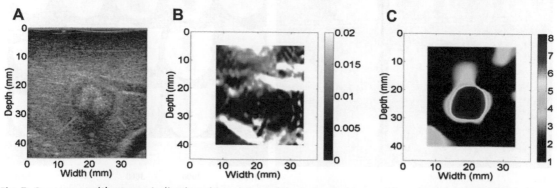

Fig. 5. Sonogram with arrows indicating ablated tissue (*A*), strain elastogram (*B*), and modulus elastogram (*C*) of RF ex vivo ablated bovine liver. (*Courtesy of* Drs T.J. Hall, T. Varghese, and J. Jiang, University of Wisconsin-Madison, Madison, WI.)

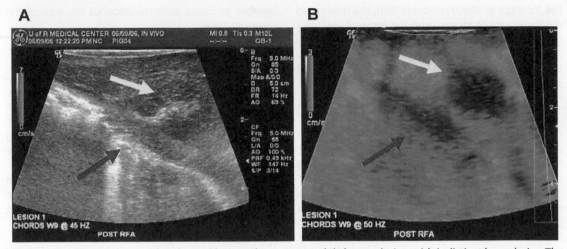

Fig. 6. In vivo porcine liver with a thermal lesion. The sonogram (*A*) shows a lesion with indistinct boundaries. The sonoelastogram (*B*) demonstrates a vibration deficit indicating a hard lesion. Yellow arrows point to the lesion. Red arrows point the boundary of the liver.

Transient Elastography Based on Arrival Time Estimation

A major limitation of harmonic elastography is that shear waves attenuate rapidly as they propagate within soft tissues, which limits the depth of penetration. The transient approach to elastography overcomes this limitation by using the acoustic radiation force of an ultrasound transducer to perturb tissue locally.[51–53] This elastographic imaging method uses an ultrasound scanner with an ultra-high frame rate (ie, 10,000 frames per second) to track the propagation of shear waves. As in harmonic elastography, local estimates of shear modulus are estimated from local estimates of wavelength. The reflections of shear waves at internal tissue boundaries make it difficult, however, to measure shear wave velocity—this limitation can be overcome by computing wave speeds directly from the arrival times, as discussed by Ji

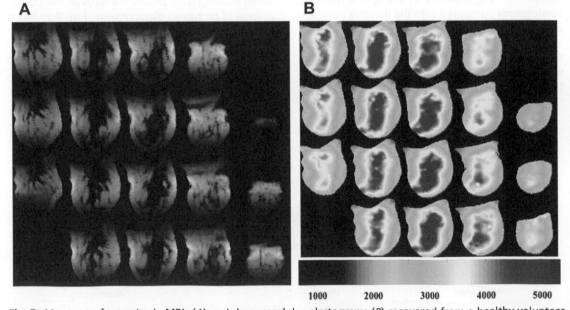

| 1000 | 2000 | 3000 | 4000 | 5000 |

Fig. 7. Montage of magnitude MRIs (*A*) and shear modulus elastograms (*B*) recovered from a healthy volunteer using the subzone inversion scheme. (*Courtesy of* Drs J.B. Weaver and K.D. Paulsen, Dartmouth College, Thayer School of Engineering, Dartmouth, NH.)

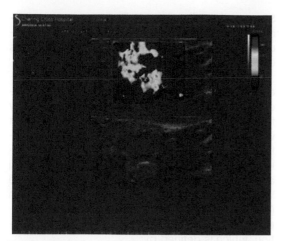

Fig. 8. Comparison transient shear wave (*upper*) and B-scan (*lower*) images of a breast with pathology confirmed IDC. The maximum diameter on the longitudinal axis on B-mode was 17 mm, whereas elastographic techniques indicated a larger footprint of the cancer. (*Courtesy of* Dr W. Svensson, Imperial College, London).

and colleagues.[54] **Fig. 8** shows an example of shear wave elastograms obtained from a breast cancer patient using a commercially available transient elastography system.

THE FUTURE OF ELASTOGRAPHY

Soft tissues display several biomechanical properties, including viscosity and nonlinearity, which may improve the diagnostic value of elastography when visualized alone or in combination with shear modulus. For example, clinicians could use mechanical nonlinearity to differentiate between benign and malignant breast tumors.[1] Furthermore, there is mounting evidence that other mechanical parameters, namely viscosity[55,56] and anisotropy,[57] could also differentiate between benign and malignant tissues—similar claims have also been made for shear modulus.[57] Not only can these mechanical parameters discriminate between different tissue types but also they may provide value in other clinical areas, including brain imaging,[58,59] distinguishing the mechanical properties of active and passive muscle groups,[60–62] characterizing blood clots,[63] and gnosing edema.[64] Several investigators are actively developing techniques to visualize different mechanical properties using quasistatic, harmonic, and transient elastographic imaging approaches.

Viscoelasticity

In most approaches to elastography, the mechanical behavior of soft tissues is modeled using the theory of linear elasticity (Hooke's law), which is an appropriate model for linear elastic materials (ie, Hookean materials). It is well known, however, that most materials, including soft tissues, deviate from Hooke's law in various ways. Materials that exhibit both fluid-like and elastic (ie, viscoelastic) mechanical behavior deviate from Hooke's law.[20] For viscoelastic materials, the relationship between stress and strain is dependent on time. Viscoelastic materials display 3 unique mechanical behaviors: (1) strain increases with time when stress (externally applied load) is sustained over a period of time, a phenomenon known as viscoelastic creep; (2) stress decreases with time when strain is held constant, a phenomenon known as viscoelastic relaxation; and (3) during cyclic loading, mechanical energy is dissipated in the form of heat, a phenomenon known as hysteresis.

Several investigators are actively developing elastographic imaging methods to visualize the mechanical parameters that characterize linear viscoelastic materials (ie, viscosity, shear modulus, and Poisson ratio). For example, Asbach and colleagues[60] developed a multifrequency method to measure the viscoelastic properties of normal liver tissue versus diseased liver tissue taken from patients with grades 3 and 4 liver fibrosis. They computed the shear modulus and viscosity variations within the tissue by fitting a Maxwell rheological model to the measured data and solving the linear viscoelastic wave equation in the frequency domain. They observed that fibrotic liver tissue had a higher viscosity (14.4 ± 6.6 Pa s) and elastic modulus (μ_1 = 2.91 ± 0.84 kPa and μ_2 = 4.83 ± 1.77 kPa) than normal liver tissue. Their results revealed that although liver tissue is dispersive, it appeared as nondispersive between the frequency range of 25 Hz to 50 Hz. Catheline and colleagues[65] computed the shear modulus (μ) and viscosity (η) by fitting the measured speed of sound and attenuation equation to Voigt and Maxwell rheological models. They observed that the recovered shear modulus values were independent of the rheological model used, but viscosity values were highly dependent on the models used.

Sinkus and colleagues[56] developed a direct-inversion scheme to visualize the mechanical properties of visocelastic materials, in which a curl operation was performed on the time-harmonic displacement field $\mathbf{u}(\mathbf{x},t) = \mathbf{u}(\mathbf{x},t)e^{i\omega t}$ to remove the displacement contribution of the compressional wave. They derived the governing equation that describes the motion incurred in an isotropic, viscoelastic medium by computing the curl of the PDEs that describe the motion incurred by both transverse and compressional shear waves. The resulting PDEs for transverse waves are given in compact form by:

$$\rho \partial_t^2 \mathbf{u} = \mu \nabla^2 \mathbf{u} + \eta \partial_t \nabla^2 \mathbf{u} \qquad (17)$$

Sinkus and colleagues[56] developed a direct-inversion scheme from Equation 17, in which μ and η were the unknowns. They evaluated the inversion scheme using (1) computer simulations, (2) phantom studies, and (3) patient studies. Their simulation studies revealed that the proposed algorithm could accurately recover shear modulus and viscosity from ideal displacement data. With noisy displacements, however, a good estimate of shear modulus was obtained only when the shear modulus of the simulated tissue was less than 8 kPa. The inversion scheme overestimated the shear modulus values when actual stiffness of the tissue was larger than 8 kPa. A similar effect was observed when estimating viscosity, albeit much earlier (ie, the algorithm provided good estimates of viscosity when $\mu < 5$ kPa). Although the shear modulus affected the bias in the viscosity measurement, the investigators demonstrated that the converse did not occur (ie, the viscosity did not affect the bias in shear modulus). Despite these issues, their phantom studies revealed that inclusions were discernible in both μ and η elastograms, and the viscosity values agreed with previously reported values for gelatin (0.21 Pa s). The patient studies revealed that the shear modulus values of malignant breast tumors were noticeably higher than those of benign fibroadenomas, but there was no significant difference observed in the viscosity of the tumor types, a result that seems to contradict results reported by Qiu and colleagues.[55]

Nonlinearity

When soft tissues deform by a small amount (an infinitesimal deformation), their geometry in the undeformed and deformed states is similar, thus the deformation is characterized using engineering strain. To characterize finite deformation, first a reference configuration has to be defined, which is the geometry of the tissue under investigation in either the deformed or undeformed state. The Green-Lagrangian strain is defined as:

$$\varepsilon_{ij} = \frac{1}{2} \left[\frac{\partial u_i}{\partial x_j} + \frac{\partial u_j}{\partial x_i} + \frac{\partial u_k}{\partial x_i} \frac{\partial u_k}{\partial x_j} \right] \qquad (18)$$

The nonlinear term is neglected when the magnitude of the spatial derivative is small, to produce the linear strain tensor, as defined in Equation 4. The relationship between stress and strain is nonlinear even for a linearly elastic material when it is undergoing finite deformations. Consequently,

Skovoroda and colleagues[66] proposed a direct-inversion scheme to reconstruct the shear modulus distribution of a linear elastic material that is undergoing finite deformation.

Some materials exhibit nonlinear material properties that are typically described using a strain energy density function. Among the strain energy functions proposed in the literature, the most widely used for modeling tissues are (1) the neo-Hookean hyperelastic model and (2) the neo-Hookean model with an exponential term. Oberai and colleagues[67] used a different model, the Veronda-Westman strain energy density function (W), to describe the finite displacement of a hyperelastic solid that is undergoing finite deformation, which is defined by:

$$W = \mu_0 \left(\frac{e^{\gamma(I_1 - 3)} - 1}{\gamma} - \frac{I_2 - 3}{2} \right) \qquad (19)$$

where the terms I_1 and I_2 are the first and second invariants of the Cauchy-Green strain tensor, μ_0 is the shear modulus, and γ denotes the nonlinearity. For the nonlinear case, they proposed an iterative inversion approach to reconstruct a nonlinear parameter and the shear modulus at zero strain.

Using data obtained from volunteer breast cancer patients, one with a benign fibroadenoma tumor and another with an invasive ductal carcinoma (IDC), Oberai and colleagues[67] observed that for the fibroadenoma case, the tumor was visible in modulus elastograms that had been computed using small strain and large strain (12%), although the contrast of the elastograms computed at large strain (7:1) was lower than that computed at smaller strain (10:1). The fibroadenoma tumor was not visible in nonlinear parameter elastograms. The inclusion in the patient with IDC was discernible in shear modulus elastograms recovered using small and large strains. The stiffness contrast of the modulus elastograms recovered at both small and large strains was comparable, however, and the IDC tumor was visible in nonlinear parameter elastograms. This result is one of several that have demonstrated the clinical value of nonlinear elastographic imaging. Specifically, elastography can characterize the nonlinear behavior of soft tissues and may be used to differentiate between benign and malignant tumors.

REFERENCES

1. Krouskop TA, Wheeler TM, Kallel F, et al. Elastic moduli of breast and prostate tissues under compression. Ultrason Imaging 1998;20:260–74.

2. Parker KJ, Doyley MM, Rubens DJ. Imaging the elastic properties of tissue: the 20 year perspective. Phys Med Biol 2011;56:R1–29.

3. Samani A, Zubovits J, Plewes D. Elastic moduli of normal and pathological human breast tissues: an inversion-technique-based investigation of 169 samples. Phys Med Biol 2007;52:1565–76.

4. Sarvazyan AP, Skovoroda AR, Emelianov SY, et al. Biophysical bases of elasticity imaging. Acoust Imaging 1995;21:223–40.

5. Lerner RM, Parker KJ, Holen J, et al. Sono-elasticity: medical elasticity images derived from ultrasound signals in mechanically vibrated targets. Acoust Imaging 1988;16:317–27.

6. O'Donnell M, Skovoroda AR, Shapo BM, et al. Internal displacement and strain imaging using ultrasonic speckle tracking. IEEE Trans Ultrason Ferroelectrics Freq Contr 1994;41(3):314–25.

7. Ophir J, Cespedes I, Ponnekanti H, et al. Elastography: a quantitative method for imaging the elasticity of biological tissues. Ultrason Imaging 1991;13:111–34.

8. Bishop J, Samani A, Sciarretta J, et al. Two-dimensional MR elastography with linear inversion reconstruction: methodology and noise analysis. Phys Med Biol 2000;45:2081–91.

9. Muthupillai R, Lomas DJ, Rossman PJ, et al. Magnetic-resonance elastography by direct visualization of propagating acoustic strain waves. Science 1995;269:1854–7.

10. Sinkus R, Lorenzen J, Schrader D, et al. High-resolution tensor MR elastography for breast tumour detection. Phys Med Biol 2000;45:1649–64.

11. Weaver JB, Van Houten EE, Miga MI, et al. Magnetic resonance elastography using 3D gradient echo measurements of steady-state motion. Med Phys 2001;28:1620–8.

12. Khalil AS, Chan RC, Chau AH, et al. Tissue elasticity estimation with optical coherence elastography: toward mechanical characterization of In vivo soft tissue. Ann Biomed Eng 2005;33:1631–9.

13. Kirkpatrick SJ, Wang RK, Duncan DD. OCT-based elastography for large and small deformations. Opt Express 2006;14:11585–97.

14. Ko HJ, Tan W, Stack R, et al. Optical coherence elastography of engineered and developing tissue. Tissue Eng 2006;12:63–73.

15. Bamber JC, Barbone PE, Bush NL, et al. Progress in freehand elastography of the breast. IEICE Trans Inf Sys 2002;E85d:5–14.

16. Greenleaf JF, Fatemi M, Insana M. Selected methods for imaging elastic properties of biological tissues. Annu Rev Biomed Eng 2003;5:57–78.

17. Manduca A, Dutt V, Borup DT, et al. Inverse approach to the calculation of elasticity maps for magnetic resonance elastography. SPIE Med Imaging Proceedings 1998;3338:426–36.

18. Ophir J, Garra B, Kallel F, et al. Elastographic imaging. Ultrasound Med Biol 2000;26(Suppl 1):S23–9.

19. Doyley MM. Model-based elastography: a survey of approaches to the inverse elasticity problem. Phys Med Biol 2012;57:R35–73.

20. Fung YC. Biomechanics: mechanical properties of living tissue. New York: Springer; 1981.

21. Timoshenko SP, Goodier JN. Theory of elasticity. Singapore: McGraw-Hill; 1970.

22. Landau LD, Lifshitz EM, Kosevich AM, et al. Theory of elasticity. Oxford (United Kingdom): Elsevier Butterworth-Heinemann; 1986.

23. Ophir J, Alam SK, Garra B, et al. Elastography: ultrasonic estimation and imaging of the elastic properties of tissues. Proc Inst Mech Eng H 1999;213:203–33.

24. Van Houten EE, Miga MI, Weaver JB, et al. Three-dimensional subzone-based reconstruction algorithm for MR elastography. Magn Reson Med 2001;45:827–37.

25. Bilgen M, Insana M. Elastostatics of a spherical inclusion in homogeneous biological media. Phys Med Biol 1998;43:1–20.

26. Kallel F, Bertrand M, Ophir J. Fundamental limitations on the contrast-transfer efficiency in elastography: an analytic study. Ultrasound Med Biol 1996;22:463–70.

27. Love A. The stress produced in a semi-infinite solid by pressure on part of the boundary. In: Philosophical transactions of the Royal Society of London, vol 228. London: The Royal Society; 1929. p. 377–420.

28. Sumi C, Suzuki A, Nakayama K. Estimation of shear modulus distribution in soft-tissue from strain distribution. IEEE Trans Biomed Eng 1995;42:193–202.

29. Brigham JC, Aquino W, Mitri FG, et al. Inverse estimation of viscoelastic material properties for solids immersed in fluids using vibroacoustic techniques. J Appl Phys 2007;101:023509–1–14.

30. Hall TJ, Bilgen M, Insana MF, et al. Phantom materials for elastography. IEEE Trans Ultrason Ferroelectrics Freq Contr 1997;44:1355–65.

31. Konofagou E, Dutta P, Ophir J, et al. Reduction of stress nonuniformities by apodization of compressor displacement in elastography. Ultrasound Med Biol 1996;22:1229–36.

32. McLaughlin J, Renzi D. Shear wave speed recovery in transient elastography and supersonic imaging using propagating fronts. Inverse Probl 2006;22:681–706.

33. Miga MI. A new approach to elastography using mutual information and finite elements. Phys Med Biol 2003;48:467–80.

34. Parker KJ, Huang SR, Musulin RA, et al. Tissue-response to mechanical vibrations for sonoelasticity imaging. Ultrasound Med Biol 1990;16:241–6.

35. Ponnekanti H, Ophir J, Cespedes I. Ultrasonic-imaging of the stress-distribution in elastic media due to an external compressor. Ultrasound Med Biol 1994;20:27–33.

36. Samani A, Bishop J, Plewes DB. A constrained modulus reconstruction technique for breast cancer assessment. IEEE Trans Med Imaging 2001; 20:877–85.

37. Bamber JC, Bush NL. Freehand elasticity imaging using speckle decorrelation rate. New York: Plenum Press; 1995.

38. Rizzatto G, Chersevani R, Solbiati L. High resolution ultrasound assists in breast diagnosis. Diagn Imaging Int 1993;9:42–5.

39. Skovoroda AR, Aglyamov SR. On reconstruction of elastic properties of soft biological tissues exposed to low-frequencies. Biofizika 1995;40:1329–34.

40. Doyley MM, Bamber JC, Shiina T, et al. Reconstruction of elasticity modulus distribution from envelope detected B-mode data. Proc IEEE Ultrason Symp 1996;2:1611–4.

41. Kallel F, Bertrand M. Tissue elasticity reconstruction using linear perturbation method. IEEE Trans Med Imaging 1996;15:299–313.

42. Doyley MM, Meaney PM, Bamber JC. Evaluation of an iterative reconstruction method for quantitative elastography. Phys Med Biol 2000;45:1521–40.

43. Jiang J, Varghese T, Brace CL, et al. Young's modulus reconstruction for radio-frequency ablation electrode-induced displacement fields: a feasibility study. IEEE Trans Med Imaging 2009; 28:1325–34.

44. Richards MS, Barbone PE, Oberai AA. Quantitative three-dimensional elasticity imaging from quasi-static deformation: a phantom study. Phys Med Biol 2009;54:757–79.

45. Yamakoshi Y, Sato J, Sato T. Ultrasonic imaging of internal vibrtation of soft tissue under forced vibration. IEEE Trans Ultrason Ferroelectrics Freq Contr 1990;37:45–53.

46. Lerner RM, Huang SR, Parker KJ. "Sonoelasticity" images derived from ultrasound signals in mechanically vibrated tissues. Ultrasound Med Biol 1990; 16:231–9.

47. Manduca A, Oliphant TE, Dresner MA, et al. Magnetic resonance elastography: non-invasive mapping of tissue elasticity. Med Image Anal 2001;5: 237–54.

48. Wu Z, Hoyt K, Rubens DJ, et al. Sonoelastographic imaging of interference patterns for estimation of shear velocity distribution in biomaterials. J Acoust Soc Am 2006;120:535–45.

49. Doyley MM, Srinivasan S, Pendergrass SA, et al. Compartive evaluation of strain-based and model-based modulus elastography. Ultrasound Med Biol 2004;31:787–802.

50. Van Houten EE, Doyley MM, Kennedy FE, et al. Initial in vivo experience with steady-state sub-zone-based MR elastography of the human breast. J Magn Reson Imaging 2003;17:72–85.

51. McAleavey S, Collins E, Kelly J, et al. Validation of SMURF estimation of shear modulus in hydrogels. Ultrason Imaging 2009;31:131–50.

52. Nightingale K, McAleavey S, Trahey G. Shear-wave generation using acoustic radiation force: in vivo and ex vivo results. Ultrasound Med Biol 2003;29: 1715–23.

53. Sarvazyan AP, Rudenko OV, Swanson SD, et al. Shear wave elasticity imaging: a new ultrasonic technology of medical diagnostics. Ultrasound Med Biol 1998;24:1419–35.

54. Ji L, McLaughlin JR, Renzi D, et al. Interior elastodynamics inverse problems: shear wave speed reconstruction in transient elastography. Inverse Probl 2003;19:S1–29.

55. Qiu YP, Sridhar M, Tsou JK, et al. Ultrasonic viscoelasticity imaging of nonpalpable breast tumors: preliminary results. Acad Radiol 2008;15: 1526–33.

56. Sinkus R, Tanter M, Xydeas T, et al. Viscoelastic shear properties of in vivo breast lesions measured by MR elastography. Magn Reson Imaging 2005; 23:159–65.

57. Sinkus R, Tanter M, Catheline S, et al. Imaging anisotropic and viscous properties of breast tissue by magnetic resonance-elastography. Magn Reson Med 2005;53:372–87.

58. Hamhaber U, Klatt D, Papazoglou S, et al. In vivo magnetic resonance elastography of human brain at 7 T and 1.5 T. J Magn Reson Imaging 2010;32: 577–83.

59. Sack I, Beierbach B, Wuerfel J, et al. The impact of aging and gender on brain viscoelasticity. Neuroimage 2009;46:652–7.

60. Asbach P, Klatt D, Hamhaber U, et al. Assessment of liver viscoelasticity using multifrequency MR elastography. Magn Reson Med 2008;60: 373–9.

61. Hoyt K, Castaneda B, Parker KJ. Two-dimensional sonoelastographic shear velocity imaging. Ultrasound Med Biol 2008;34:276–88.

62. Perrinez PR, Kennedy FE, Van Houten EE, et al. Modeling of soft poroelastic tissue in time-harmonic MR elastography. IEEE Trans Biomed Eng 2009;56:598–608.

63. Schmitt C, Soulez G, Maurice RL, et al. Noninvasive vascular elastography: toward a complementary characterization tool of atherosclerosis in carotid arteries. Ultrasound Med Biol 2007;33: 1841–58.

64. Righetti R, Garra BS, Mobbs LM, et al. The feasibility of using poroelastographic techniques for

distinguishing between normal and lymphedematous tissues in vivo. Phys Med Biol 2007;52: 6525–41.

65. Catheline S, Gennisson J, Delon G, et al. Measurement of viscoelastic properties of homogeneous soft solid using transient elastography: an inverse problem approach. J Acoust Soc Am 2004;116: 3734–41.

66. Skovoroda AR, Lubinski MA, Emelianov SY, et al. Reconstructive elasticity imaging for large deformations. IEEE Trans Ultrason Ferroelectrics Freq Contr 1999;46:523–35.

67. Oberai AA, Gokhale NH, Goenezen S, et al. Linear and nonlinear elasticity imaging of soft tissue in vivo: demonstration of feasibility. Phys Med Biol 2009;54:1191–207.

Elastography of Thyroid Masses

Manjiri K. Dighe, MD

KEYWORDS

- Elastography • Thyroid • Papillary carcinoma • Nodule

KEY POINTS

- Techniques of elastography are available to evaluate the thyroid nodule.
- Many reasons exist for false positive and false negative results in elastography.
- Appropriate use of elastography is an adjunct to ultrasound and not a replacement.

DISCUSSION OF PROBLEM/CLINICAL PRESENTATION

The prevalence of thyroid nodules is approximately 3% to 8% in the general population[1–4] but increases to almost 50% after 65 years of age.[5] With advances in technology, incidence of thyroid nodules on ultrasound (US) has increased to almost 60%; however, the incidence of malignancy in thyroid is low at 5% to 15%.[6,7] In addition, B-mode and Doppler US have been found to have low accuracy. Fine needle aspiration (FNA) is the standard procedure to determine if a nodule is cancerous or not; however, FNA is an invasive procedure and would result in an inadequate sample in 10% to 20% of cases leading to rebiopsy.[6] Palpation has been used in clinical examination to assess if a thyroid nodule is firm or palpable; however, palpation is subjective and will vary depending on the size and location of the nodule.[8]

IMAGING PROTOCOLS
Imaging Findings

US elastography is a promising new technique in the evaluation of the thyroid nodule. It allows for "virtual palpation" of the nodule, which may not be otherwise palpable. US elastography was developed to obtain information on tissue stiffness noninvasively.[9–11] Due to the superficial location of the thyroid gland, it is feasible to obtain information regarding the stiffness in the organ or nodule.

Most malignant tumors are characterized by the presence of abnormally firm stroma due to the presence of collagen and myofibroblasts, which is the desmoplastic transformation. This tumor stroma promotes the proliferation of malignant cells (and could even initiate them).[12] However, certain benign fibrous tumors can be very stiff as well (histiocytofibromas, for example). Previous ex vivo studies had suggested that there is considerable difference between the stiffness in normal thyroid tissue and thyroid tumors.[13,14] Based on this observation, multiple in vivo studies were then performed to differentiate benign from malignant thyroid nodules. Various techniques exist for performing elastography as outlined in the other articles. A brief description of these techniques and their utility in thyroid elastography are mentioned here.

Quasi-static or strain elastography or sonoelastography

In quasi-static or strain elastography, the US probe is placed on the neck with gel interposition and compression is generated by pressure applied by the operator with the US probe on the skin. Improvement in the sensitivity of very small tissue movement detection has made it possible to use

Funding Sources: The author has received funding from NIH, R21 (Thyroid Elastography).
Department of Radiology, University of Washington, Seattle, WA 98195, USA
E-mail address: dighe@uw.edu

ultrasound.theclinics.com

carotid pulsation to induce this tissue deformation.[15] Classification using 4 or 5 visual categorical scores (**Figs. 1** and **2**), either color coded or in gray scale, has been proposed.[16] Semi-quantitative analysis provides numerical values that correspond to the deformation ratios. The machine calculates a ratio between the zones of interest (regions of interest [ROI]) placed by the operator on the nodule and on the healthy tissue. The calculation can thus be made using the rates of deformation of the structure ("strain rate") (**Figs. 3** and **4**).[17]

A recent meta-analysis by Bojunga and colleagues,[18] which included 639 nodules, reported a mean sensitivity of 92% and a specificity of 90% using strain elastography for the diagnosis of malignant thyroid nodules; however, the patient population was highly selected with a 24% prevalence of malignancy and many patients were sent to surgery.

Two recent studies[19,20] with 309 and 97 patients, respectively, used strain values and ratios to determine thyroid nodule stiffness. All patients were referred to surgery. Vorländer and colleagues[19] used a proprietary absolute measurement of strain value, which ranged from 1.0 (maximum soft) to 0.1 (maximum hard) and reported a negative predictive value (NPV) for malignancy of 100% using a strain ratio cutoff of greater than 0.31 and a positive predictive value (PPV) of 42% using a cutoff of less than 0.15. Cantisani and colleagues[20] reported a sensitivity, specificity, PPV, and NPV of 97.3%, 91.7%, 87.8%, and 98.2%, respectively, for the prediction

of malignancy using a strain ratio ≥ 2 (ratio of lesion strain to surrounding parenchyma). Elastography was more sensitive and specific than all conventional US features.

Another study compared strain elastography based on 4 point scores and the strain ratios between the nodule and the surrounding thyroid at the same depth.[21] The diagnostic accuracy of the strain ratio evaluation was slightly higher (0.88 vs 0.79, $P<.001$) than that of the elastography score, with a higher specificity. Another prospective study[22] evaluated strain elastography in 51 patients with small single solid nodules of 3 to 10 mm submitted to surgical resection. The 5-point scale developed by Itoh and colleagues[16] for the breast elastography was used in this study; with a cutoff at 3/4, a sensitivity of 91%, specificity of 89%, PPV 94%, and NPV 85% for the diagnosis of malignant nodules was found. Thus, strain elastography seems to have a potential even in small nodules.

However, additional studies, including only a few follicular carcinomas, revealed inconclusive data on the value of elastography. Most malignant nodules missed by elastography were follicular carcinomas, which can be soft and difficult to differentiate from benign nodules.[18] Strain elastography was evaluated in 102 patients with indeterminate cytology who went to surgery.[23] Histology revealed 64 follicular adenomas, 32 follicular variants of papillary thyroid cancer, 4 follicular carcinomas, and 2 hyperplastic nodules. In this selected population, strain elastography (4-point scale) only reached a PPV of 34% and an NPV

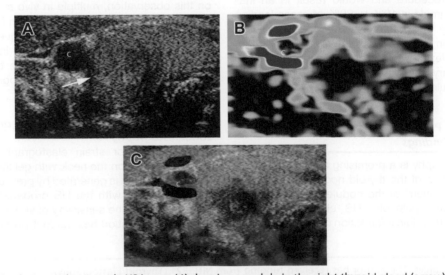

Fig. 1. Strain elastography: B-mode US image (*A*) showing a nodule in the right thyroid gland (*arrow*). This lesion showed increased stiffness on elastography (*B*) and the overlay image (*color overlayed on B-mode*) (*C*) with predominantly blue color (high stiffness), which was shown to be a follicular adenoma on histopathology. C, carotid artery.

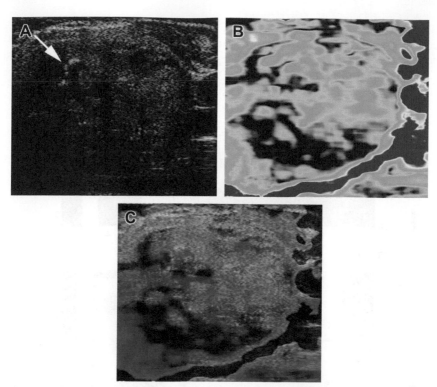

Fig. 2. Strain elastography: B-mode US image (*A*) showing a nodule in the left thyroid gland with small areas of calcification in it (*arrow*). This lesion showed increased stiffness on elastography (*B*) and the overlay image (*color overlayed* on B-mode) (*C*) with a combination of blue and green color (moderate stiffness), which was shown to be a papillary carcinoma on histopathology.

of 50%. Conversely, Cantisani and colleagues[24] reported a study including 140 nodules with indeterminate cytology in which elastography with a strain ratio greater than 2.05 achieved sensitivity, specificity, NPV, PPV, and accuracy of 87.5%, 92%, 94.8%, 81.4%, 89.8%, respectively.

Acoustic radiation force imaging

In acoustic radiation force imaging (ARFI), an ROI is placed in the thyroid nodule while performing real-time B-mode imaging. The tissue at the ROI is mechanically excited using acoustic pulses to generate localized tissue displacements. These displacements result in shear-wave propagation away from the region of excitation and are tracked using ultrasonic, correlation-based methods.[25] The maximum displacement is estimated for many US tracking beams and the shear wave speed of the tissue can be reconstructed[26,27] along with the shear wave propagation velocity. Because there is no mechanical or external pressure used in ARFI and because shear wave propagation velocity is proportional to the square root of tissue elasticity, stiffness of the nodule can be calculated.[28]

A study by Bojunga and colleagues[28] found that the median velocity of ARFI imaging in the healthy

thyroid tissue, benign and malignant thyroid nodules was 1.76 m/s, 1.90 m/s, and 2.69 m/s, respectively. They did not find any significant difference in median velocity between healthy thyroid tissue and benign thyroid nodules; however, a significant difference was found between malignant thyroid nodules and healthy thyroid tissue and malignant thyroid nodules and benign thyroid nodules. A study by Azizi and colleagues[29] found that the NPV of ARFI was better than the PPV; however, the PPV of ARFI was better than that of B-mode criteria of hypoechogenicity. Gu and colleagues[30] in their study found that ARFI had a high sensitivity and specificity in evaluating benign and malignant nodules when they used a cutoff value of 2.555 m/s. Sporea and colleagues[31] used ARFI in evaluating the utility of ARFI in diffuse thyroid disease. They found that the optimal cutoff value for the prediction of diffuse thyroid pathologic abnormality with ARFI was 2.36 m/s, which had a sensitivity of 62.5%, specificity of 79.5%, PPV of 87.6%, NPV of 55.5%, and accuracy of 72.7%.

Shear wave elastography

Shear wave elastography (SWE) is a user-independent method with no compressive fertilization is a risk factor for accreta.[9] All of these have in common a potential defect in the decidua basalis. Nulliparous women with placenta previa have a risk of accreta of 1% to 3%, whereas those with 2 or more prior cesareans and a placenta previa or low-lying anterior placenta increase their risk of accreta to 30% to 50%.[2] An unusual risk factor that has been suggested is prior chemotherapy for gestational trophoblastic disease.[10] The highest rates of creta are reported from Thailand, and it has been postulated that this may relate to the higher rates of gestational trophoblastic disease in the Far East.[11] A case of percreta in a patient with prior pelvic irradiation has been reported.[12] Another case of accreta has been attributed to a myometrial defect that occurred subsequent to uterine artery embolization for a symptomatic leiomyoma.[13] The articles describing these case reports advise imaging to evaluate for accreta as part of the antenatal care in women with prior uterine artery embolization.[13]

Treatment of placenta creta is best accomplished in centers that have the expertise to handle the management, which involves multiple disciplines, including blood bank, interventional radiology, anesthesia, and surgical expertise—gynecologic oncology, urology, or obstetric subspecialty expertise. In a retrospective study, Eller and colleagues[14] found that maternal morbidity, including large-volume blood transfusion, reoperation within 7 days, and other complications, was reduced in women with accreta treated in tertiary care hospitals with multidisciplinary teams compared with women with accreta who received standard obstetric care.

More recently, attempts at conservative (uterine preservation) management have become more frequent, although many of the more severe cases do come to hysterectomy. In a retrospective multi-center study of tertiary university hospitals caring for women with creta, outcomes for conservative management, defined as leaving the placenta in situ, partially or entirely, without attempts at forceful removal, was evaluated.[15] The primary outcome was uterine conservation, with secondary outcomes a composite of the various potential severe maternal morbidities. Conservative therapy was found successful in 78.4%, with 10.8% each undergoing primary hysterectomy and delayed hysterectomy. Severe maternal morbidity, defined as including infections, fistulas, injuries to adjacent organs, thrombotic episodes, acute pulmonary edema, or acute renal failure, occurred in 6% of cases. Higher rates of maternal morbidity were seen with placenta percreta, particularly with bladder involvement. The investigators speculated that conservative therapy for percreta with bladder involvement may avoid

some of the urologic complications that have been described, including bladder lacerations and fistulas, transected ureters, and small residual bladder capacity due to partial cystectomy.

ETIOLOGY OF PLACENTA ACCRETA

There are three main postulated etiologies for placenta accreta, which may separately or together come into play in this condition; deficient decidua, overinvasiveness of trophoblast,[1] and alterations in maternal vascularity.[16] Probably the least touted theory is that of vascular alterations as the primary cause. There has been some evidence that there are differences in angiogenic growth factors and their receptors in placenta accreta.[16] Tseng and colleagues postulate that these may relate to the uteroplacental neovascularization seen with placenta accreta.

Increased trophoblast invasiveness is another theory of the origin of placenta creta, although that is not subscribed to by all investigators. Cohen and colleagues[17] reported that the cytotrophoblast, but not the decidua, has a major role in cytotrophoblast invasiveness, secreting factors, such as matrix metalloproteinases, that increase invasiveness in vitro. They related increased invasiveness to trophoblastic disease and decreased invasiveness to preeclampsia and intrauterine growth retardation.

It has been suggested that accreta arises from an abnormal interaction between the trophoblast and the maternal tissues[18] and that there are abundant extravillous trophoblast cells present but limited placental-site giant cells in placenta accreta (Fig. 1). Abnormalities of spiral arteries have been observed, with physiologic changes deep in the myometrium but absent more superficially.[18] Deeper but defective vascular remodeling by trophoblast, as well as increased invasiveness of trophoblast into the myometrium, has been suggested as contributing to creta.[3] More recent studies have evaluated differential staining with decorin and biglycan, proteoglycans associated with cellular proliferation, migration, and invasion in the extravillous trophoblast in accreta and in invasive moles/choriocarcinomas compared with normal pregnancy, supporting increased invasiveness of the trophoblast.[7]

An in vitro study of decidual-trophoblast interactions showed that induced decidual injury by incision increases the invasive potential of trophoblasts compared with intact decidua, suggesting a combined role of abnormal or deficient decidua and increased invasiveness of trophoblast.[19] Repair of the incised decidua reversed this invasiveness in

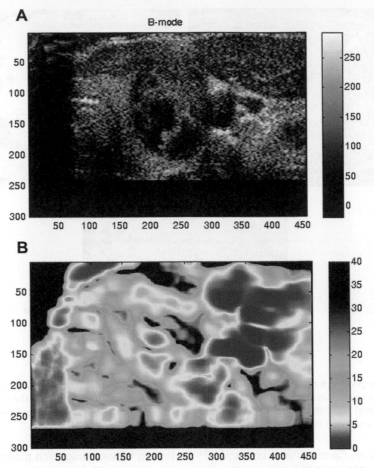

Fig. 3. Quantitative strain elastography: B-mode US image (*A*) showing a nodule in the left thyroid gland with cystic changes in it. ROIs were drawn on the lesion and adjacent to the carotid artery as shown in the elastography image (*B*). This lesion showed increased stiffness and had a thyroid stiffness index of 35, which was shown to be a papillary carcinoma on histopathology.

maneuvers needed. This methodology captures the waves that propagate from the stimulated tissue in question with an ultrafast US tracking method, which displays real-time information in terms of velocity or estimated tissue stiffness expressed in kilopascals (**Figs. 5** and **6**). Sebag and colleagues[32] reported that significantly higher elasticity index was noted in malignant thyroid nodules than benign nodules, and they reported the sensitivity and specificity of SWE were 85.2% and 93.9% using a cutoff level of 65 kPa. They reported higher diagnostic performance with a combined score (SWE+B-mode US) than that of B-mode US only. Other SWE studies[33] showed variable cutoff values yielding a maximum sum of diagnostic performance to predict thyroid malignancy. Kim and colleagues[34] in their study found similar results as the prior studies. Veyrieres and colleagues[35] were able to confirm that the cutoff value of 66 kPa was the best US sign to rule out

malignant thyroid nodules; however, they suggested that more work needed to be performed in calcified nodules and follicular tumors (**Fig. 7**).

PEARLS, PITFALLS, AND VARIANTS

Elastography provides information about the stiffness in a particular tissue similar to what palpation of a lesion would do. Most malignant tumors have abnormally firm stroma because of the presence of collagen and myofibroblasts. This desmoplastic transformation promotes the proliferation of malignant cells (and could even initiate them).[12] However, certain benign fibrous tumors can be very stiff as well (histiocytofibromas, for example). Thyroid US elastography could therefore make it possible to identify cancers with increased stiffness, such as papillary cancers; on the other hand, cancers with nonmodified elasticities will not be detected, as is the case in most follicular

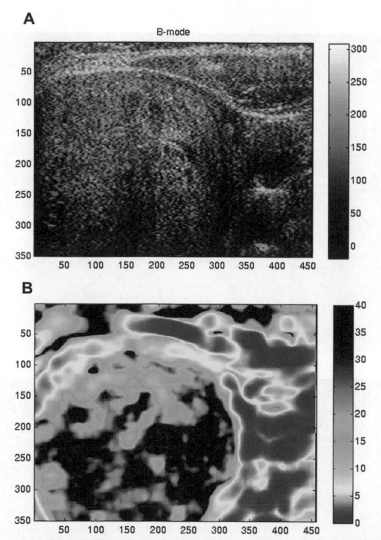

Fig. 4. Quantitative strain elastography: B-mode US image (*A*) showing a solid nodule in the left thyroid gland. ROIs were drawn on the lesion and adjacent to the carotid artery as shown in the elastography image (*B*). This lesion showed intermediate stiffness and had a thyroid stiffness index of 13.5, which was shown to be a follicular lesion with low probability of malignancy on cytology.

carcinomas (**Fig. 8**) and benign lesions with increased stiffness will fall into the false positive group with elastography (**Fig. 9**).

Quasi-static elastography was first used and involved compression of tissue manually with the transducer. This compression would bring in variability in the amount of compression applied. To overcome this variability, machines then had a mechanism to show the amount of compression applied (mild, moderate, too much) on a scale displayed in real time on the image. Currently, the improvement in the sensitivity of very small tissue movement detection makes it possible to use the carotid pulsation to induce tissue deformation.[36] Some of the limitations of quasi-static elastography include the need for an area of healthy tissue to be included in the elastography image, to be able to compare normal thyroid with the nodule. If all of the tissue in the image is abnormal, the nodule stiffness will vary with the obtained data, which could be a challenge especially in the case of a nodule in a background of an autoimmune thyroid disease.[37] Similarly if the whole thyroid lobe is involved by a large nodule, there would not be any normal thyroid to compare. Tissue elasticity data obtained from ARFI are not translated in color-coded images as in other elastography methods and this method seems to be a transition technology from strain elastography to SWE.

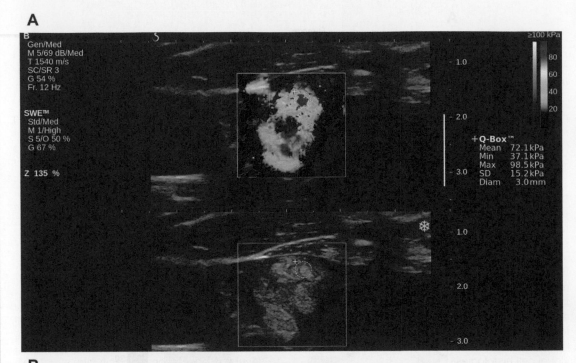

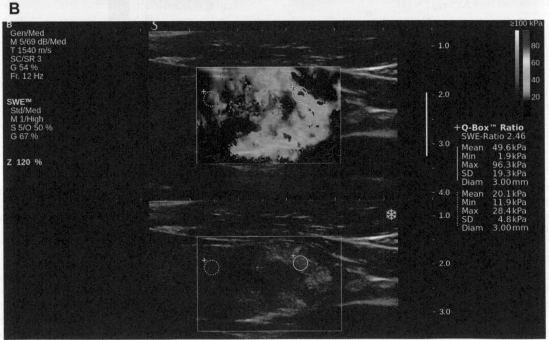

Fig. 5. SWE showing a nodule with an SWE value of 72 kPa on a transverse image (*A*) and an SWE ratio with the surrounding normal thyroid gland on the sagittal image (*B*) of 2.46, which was shown to be a papillary carcinoma in histopathology.

Intralesional calcifications are common in thyroid nodules and may bias the stiffness of the lesion, as has been shown for nodules with peripheral calcifications.[13,38,39] Elastography should also be interpreted with caution in extensive cystic areas because this may cause artifacts because of a loss of signal in the cystic region. Elastography shows high sensitivity, specificity, and NPV for the diagnosis of papillary carcinoma, which are known to be stiffer; however, the evaluations were performed in highly specialized centers with high incidences of carcinoma and data in follicular

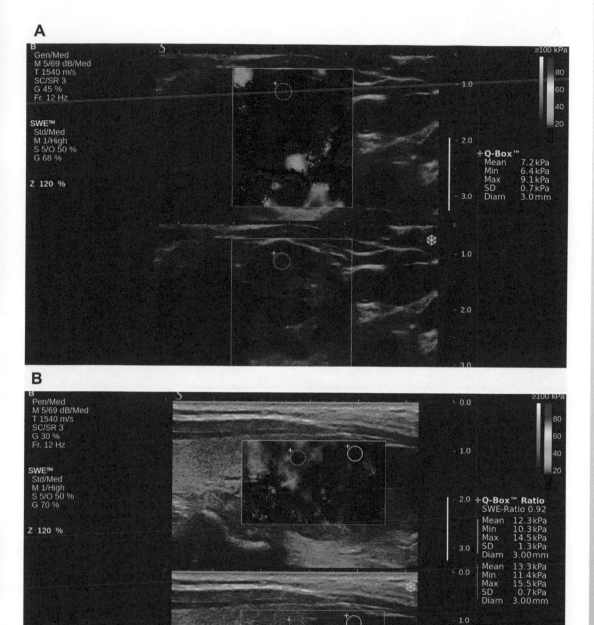

Fig. 6. SWE showing a nodule with an SWE value of 7.2 kPa on a transverse image (*A*) and an SWE ratio with the surrounding normal thyroid gland on the sagittal image (*B*) of 0.92, which was shown to be a multinodular goiter on histopathology.

carcinomas, which are softer malignancies, have not been impressive.

A recent study using strain elastography, however, reported no additional value of elastography to experienced B-mode US.[40]

WHAT THE REFERRING PHYSICIAN NEEDS TO KNOW

A recent guideline published by the European Federation of Societies for Ultrasound in Medicine

A

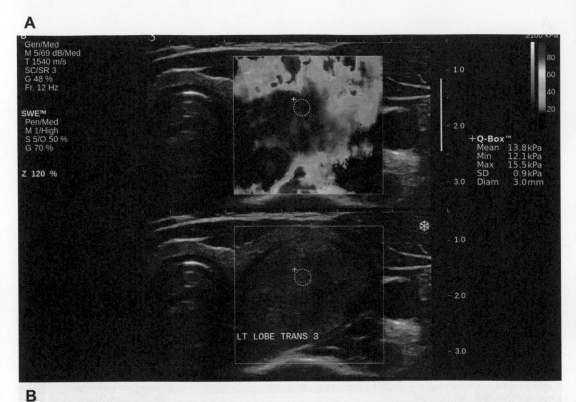

B

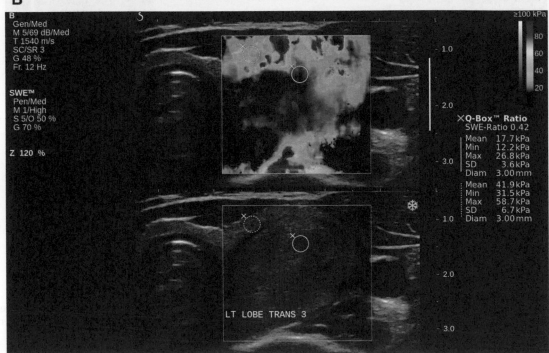

Fig. 7. SWE showing a nodule with an SWE value of 13.8 kPa on a transverse image (*A*) and an SWE ratio with the surrounding normal thyroid gland on the sagittal image (*B*) of 0.42, which was shown to be a follicular adenoma on histopathology.

A

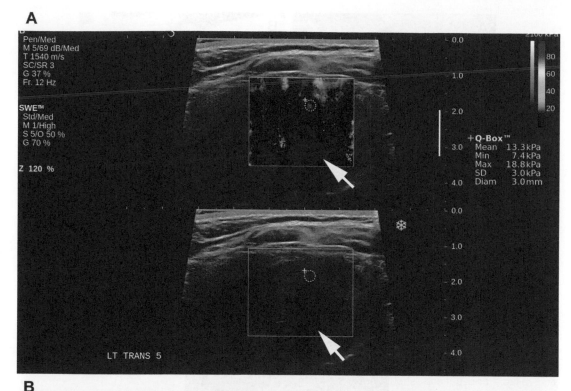

B

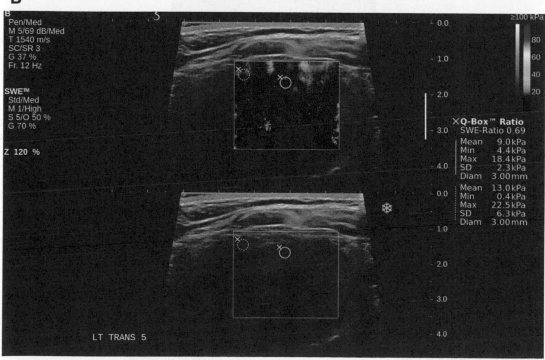

Fig. 8. SWE showing a nodule with an SWE value of 13.3 kPa on a transverse image (*A*) and an SWE ratio with the surrounding normal thyroid gland on the transverse image (*B*) of 0.69, which was shown to be a follicular carcinoma on histopathology. Note the lack of shear wave information from the deeper part of the nodule (*arrow*) due to the presence of cystic areas.

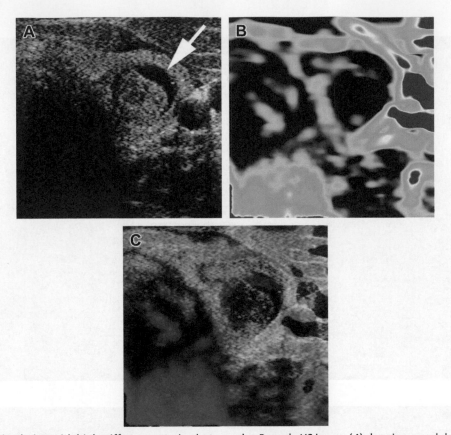

Fig. 9. Benign lesion with high stiffness on strain elastography: B-mode US image (*A*) showing a nodule in the left thyroid gland with cystic change in it (*arrow*). This lesion showed increased stiffness on elastography (*B*) and the overlay image (*color overlayed* on B-mode) (*C*) with predominantly blue color (high stiffness), which was shown to be a fibrotic nodule on histopathology.

and Biology suggests that "elastography of thyroid lesions can be performed using either strain or shear wave elastography with many high-end systems using linear transducers. No patient preparation is required." They recommend that "Elastography be used as an additional tool for thyroid lesion differentiation and based on expert opinion, elastography may be used to guide follow up of lesions negative for malignancy at FNA."[41] Elastography makes it possible to improve the PPV and the NPV of malignancy obtained from conventional US studies.[20,42] The French Endocrinology Society recently specified in its "Consensus on the treatment of thyroid nodules" that elastography must therefore be integrated as a parameter of the US classification of the nodule; however, presently, it cannot replace it in any case.

SUMMARY

Elastography is undeniably a major technological advance in thyroid imaging in recent years. The anatomic characteristics of the thyroid (superficial

organ) and the frequency of nodules in the thyroid make it an ideal organ for this technique. Static elastography is currently available in many machines. SWE is becoming the reference technique for thyroid; however, prospective studies (ongoing) will need to be performed before its routine use in the clinic. Elastography should not be considered as an alternative to conventional US, but like an additional parameter that optimizes the US imaging.[43]

REFERENCES

1. Wiest PW, Hartshorne MF, Inskip PD, et al. Thyroid palpation versus high-resolution thyroid ultrasonography in the detection of nodules. J Ultrasound Med 1998;17(8):487–96.
2. Tomimori E, Pedrinola F, Cavaliere H, et al. Prevalence of incidental thyroid disease in a relatively low iodine intake area. Thyroid 1995;5(4):273–6.
3. Carroll BA. Asymptomatic thyroid nodules: incidental sonographic detection. AJR Am J Roentgenol 1982;138(3):499–501.

4. Brander A, Viikinkoski P, Nickels J, et al. Thyroid gland: US screening in a random adult population. Radiology 1991;181(3):683–7.

5. Mortensen JD, Woolner LB, Bennett WA. Gross and microscopic findings in clinically normal thyroid glands. J Clin Endocrinol Metab 1955;15(10): 1270–80.

6. Gharib H, Goellner JR. Fine-needle aspiration biopsy of the thyroid: an appraisal. Ann Intern Med 1993;118(4):282–9.

7. Hegedüs L. Clinical practice. The thyroid nodule. N Engl J Med 2004;351(17):1764–71.

8. Tan GH, Gharib H, Reading CC. Solitary thyroid nodule. Comparison between palpation and ultrasonography. Arch Intern Med 1995;155(22):2418–23.

9. Ophir J, Alam SK, Garra B, et al. Elastography: ultrasonic estimation and imaging of the elastic properties of tissues. Proc Inst Mech Eng H 1999;213(3): 203–33.

10. Gao L, Parker KJ, Lerner RM, et al. Imaging of the elastic properties of tissue–a review. Ultrasound Med Biol 1996;22(8):959–77.

11. Greenleaf JF, Fatemi M, Insana M. Selected methods for imaging elastic properties of biological tissues. Annu Rev Biomed Eng 2003;5:57–78.

12. Mai KT, Perkins DG, Yazdi HM, et al. Infiltrating papillary thyroid carcinoma: review of 134 cases of papillary carcinoma. Arch Pathol Lab Med 1998; 122(2):166–71.

13. Rago T, Santini F, Scutari M, et al. Elastography: new developments in ultrasound for predicting malignancy in thyroid nodules. J Clin Endocrinol Metab 2007;92(8):2917–22.

14. Lyshchik A, Higashi T, Asato R, et al. Elastic moduli of thyroid tissues under compression. Ultrason Imaging 2005;27(2):101–10.

15. Dighe M, Bae U, Richardson ML, et al. Differential diagnosis of thyroid nodules with US elastography using carotid artery pulsation. Radiology 2008; 248(2):662–9.

16. Itoh A, Ueno E, Tohno E, et al. Breast disease: clinical application of US elastography for diagnosis. Radiology 2006;239(2):341–50.

17. Luo S, Kim E, Dighe M, et al. Screening of thyroid nodules by ultrasound elastography using diastolic strain variation. Conf Proc IEEE Eng Med Biol Soc 2009;1:4420–3.

18. Bojunga J, Herrmann E, Meyer G, et al. Real-time elastography for the differentiation of benign and malignant thyroid nodules: a meta-analysis. Thyroid 2010;20(10):1145–50.

19. Vorländer C, Wolff J, Saalabian S, et al. Real-time ultrasound elastography–a noninvasive diagnostic procedure for evaluating dominant thyroid nodules. Langenbecks Arch Surg 2010;395(7):865–71.

20. Cantisani V, D'Andrea V, Biancari F, et al. Prospective evaluation of multiparametric ultrasound and quantitative elastosonography in the differential diagnosis of benign and malignant thyroid nodules: preliminary experience. Eur J Radiol 2012;81(10): 2678–83.

21. Ning CP, Jiang SQ, Zhang T, et al. The value of strain ratio in differential diagnosis of thyroid solid nodules. Eur J Radiol 2012;81(2):286–91.

22. Wang Y, Dan HJ, Dan HY, et al. Differential diagnosis of small single solid thyroid nodules using real-time ultrasound elastography. J Int Med Res 2010;38(2): 466–72.

23. Lippolis PV, Tognini S, Materazzi G, et al. Is elastography actually useful in the presurgical selection of thyroid nodules with indeterminate cytology? J Clin Endocrinol Metab 2011;96(11):E1826–30.

24. Cantisani V, Ulisse S, Guaitoli E, et al. Q-elastography in the presurgical diagnosis of thyroid nodules with indeterminate cytology. PLoS One 2012;7(11): e50725.

25. Nightingale K, Nightingale R, Stutz D, et al. Acoustic radiation force impulse imaging of in vivo vastus medialis muscle under varying isometric load. Ultrason Imaging 2002;24(2):100–8.

26. Nightingale K, Zhai L, Dahl J, et al. Shear wave velocity estimation using acoustic radiation force impulsive excitation in liver in vivo. Proc 2006 IEEE Ultrasonics Symposium (IEEE). Piscataway, NJ: IEEE Operations center; 2006. p. 1156–60.

27. Kasai C, Namekawa K, Koyano A, et al. Real-time two-dimensional blood flow imaging using an autocorrelation technique. IEEE Trans Son Ultrason 1985;32:458–64.

28. Bojunga J, Dauth N, Berner C, et al. Acoustic radiation force impulse imaging for differentiation of thyroid nodules. PLoS One 2012;7(8):e42735.

29. Azizi G, Keller J, Lewis M, et al. Performance of elastography for the evaluation of thyroid nodules: a prospective study. Thyroid 2013;23(6):734–40.

30. Gu J, Du L, Bai M, et al. Preliminary study on the diagnostic value of acoustic radiation force impulse technology for differentiating between benign and malignant thyroid nodules. J Ultrasound Med 2012; 31(5):763–71.

31. Sporea I, Vlad M, Bota S, et al. Thyroid stiffness assessment by acoustic radiation force impulse elastography (ARFI). Ultraschall Med 2011;32(3): 281–5.

32. Sebag F, Vaillant-Lombard J, Berbis J, et al. Shear wave elastography: a new ultrasound imaging mode for the differential diagnosis of benign and malignant thyroid nodules. J Clin Endocrinol Metab 2010;95(12):5281–8.

33. Bhatia KS, Tong CS, Cho CC, et al. Shear wave elastography of thyroid nodules in routine clinical practice: preliminary observations and utility for detecting malignancy. Eur Radiol 2012;22(11): 2397–406.

34. Kim H, Kim JA, Son EJ, et al. Quantitative assessment of shear-wave ultrasound elastography in thyroid nodules: diagnostic performance for predicting malignancy. Eur Radiol 2013; 23(9):2532–7.

35. Veyrieres JB, Albarel F, Lombard JV, et al. A threshold value in shear wave elastography to rule out malignant thyroid nodules: a reality? Eur J Radiol 2012;81(12):3965–72.

36. Bae U, Dighe M, Dubinsky T, et al. Ultrasound thyroid elastography using carotid artery pulsation - preliminary study. J Ultrasound Med 2007;26(6): 797–805.

37. Di Pasquale M, Rothstein JL, Palazzo JP. Pathologic features of Hashimoto's-associated papillary thyroid carcinomas. Hum Pathol 2001;32(1):24–30.

38. Hong Y, Liu X, Li Z, et al. Real-time ultrasound elastography in the differential diagnosis of benign and malignant thyroid nodules. J Ultrasound Med 2009; 28(7):861–7.

39. Kim JK, Baek JH, Lee JH, et al. Ultrasound elastography for thyroid nodules: a reliable study? Ultrasound Med Biol 2012;38(9):1508–13.

40. Moon HJ, Kim EK, Yoon JH, et al. Clinical implication of elastography as a prognostic factor of papillary thyroid microcarcinoma. Ann Surg Oncol 2012; 19(7):2279–87.

41. Cosgrove D, Piscaglia F, Bamber J, et al. EFSUMB guidelines and recommendations on the clinical use of ultrasound elastography. Part 2: clinical applications. Ultraschall Med 2013;34(3):238–53.

42. Russ G, Bienvenu-Perrard M, Royer B, et al. Prospective evaluation of thyroid imaging reporting and data system on 4550 nodules with and without elastography. Eur J Endocrinol 2011;168(5):649–55.

43. Leenhardt L, Borson-Chazot F, Calzada M, et al. Good practice guide for cervical ultrasound scan and echo-guided techniques in treating differentiated thyroid cancer of vesicular origin. Ann Endocrinol (Paris) 2011;72(3):173–97.

The Special Contribution of Contrast-Enhanced Ultrasound to Oncology

Stephanie R. Wilson, MD*

KEYWORDS

- Microbubble contrast agents • Contrast-enhanced ultrasound (CEUS)
- Liver tumors: hepatocellular carcinoma, metastases, cholangiocarcinoma
- Kidney tumors: solid and cystic renal cell carcinoma • Cirrhotic liver nodules

KEY POINTS

- Real-time contrast-enhanced ultrasound (CEUS) shows vascular enhancement regardless of its timing or duration.
- Microbubble contrast agents are purely vascular and do not pass into the tumor interstitium, allowing a true depiction of tumor vascularity.
- Washout of contrast agent in the liver, after arterial-phase enhancement, has a high association with malignancy.
- Timing of washout is generally discriminatory as to the cell of origin of tumors in the liver: hepatocyte or nonhepatocyte origin.
- CEUS plays an essential role in the multimodality approach to nodules in a cirrhotic liver.
- Monitoring of ablative therapies with CEUS is effective and repeatable, reducing the requirement for repeat therapy sessions.

PREAMBLE

From a historical perspective, routine sonography has played an essential role in the surveillance of patients with a variety of symptoms and is often the first modality to detect evidence of malignant disease. Once detected, however, CT and MR imaging scan are most often chosen for further work-up, diagnosis, staging, and therapy planning for those patients ultimately proved to have malignant disease. There are a variety of reasons for this, including the inferior performance of conventional ultrasound (US) compared with contrast-enhanced CT (CECT) and contrast-enhanced magnetic resonance (CEMR) scan for tumor imaging. Furthermore, conventional Doppler imaging, although it nicely shows rapidly flowing blood in larger arteries, is unable to show blood flow at the capillary level, making comparison of routine US with CECT and CEMR unreasonable.

The most exciting advancement for US in the past 2 decades, however, has been the introduction of microbubble contrast agents, which allow, for the first time, vascular imaging with US, showing blood flow at the perfusion level and improving the already excellent large vessel vascular imaging afforded with Doppler imaging.[1] Contrast-enhanced ultrasound (CEUS) is a rapidly growing technique that uses microbubble contrast agents, which are unique in that they interact with the imaging technique, oscillating in response to exposure to a US field and disrupting when exposed to high energy, with the production of a brief but bright signal. Their growing use has transformed the role of US in the evaluation of oncology

University of Calgary, Alberta, Canada
* Department of Diagnostic Imaging, Division of Ultrasound, Foothills Medical Centre, 1403 29 Street NW, Calgary, AB Canada T2N 2T9
E-mail address: stephanie.wilson@albertahealthservices.ca

Ultrasound Clin 9 (2014) 25–41
http://dx.doi.org/10.1016/j.cult.2013.08.006
1556-858X/14/$ – see front matter © 2014 Elsevier Inc. All rights reserved.

patients, allowing US to play an essential role in the multimodality characterization of many tumors in the solid and the hollow organs.[2] CEUS has also greatly improved tumor detection capability.[3] Microbubble contrast agents have distinct advantages over those used for CT and MR imaging scan in that they are purely intravascular, thereby providing the most accurate display of the vascularity of a tumor over time.[4] CT and MR imaging contrast, by comparison have a well-recognized interstitial phase because the contrast agents can pass freely through the tumor vascular endothelium. This has the potential to mask the observation of washout of contrast as an indicator of malignant disease.[5] Furthermore, microbubble contrast agents are not nephrotoxic, they require no ionizing radiation, and their real-time evaluation provides the most accurate evaluation of enhancement regardless of its timing or duration.

The liver, in particular, has enjoyed the most intense success from CEUS because characterization of focal liver masses comprises the most common approval indication for microbubble contrast agents, worldwide.

CEUS: THE PROCEDURE

CEUS is performed with the intravenous injection of a microbubble contrast agent, comprising a perfluorocarbon gas with a supporting lipid shell. In North America, the most frequent agent to date has been Definity (Lantheus Medical Imaging, Billerica, Massachusetts). All images in this article are created using Definity. Agents have low toxicity, with severe reactions occurring with a rate of 0.001%, with no deaths in a series of more than 23,000 patients from a European cumulative experience.[6] Imaging the microbubbles

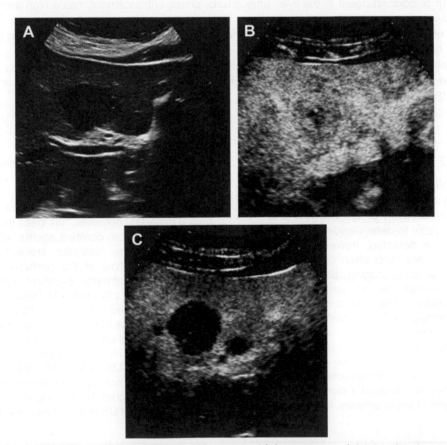

Fig. 1. The value of showing washout. A 61-year-old woman with breast cancer. (*A*) A baseline image of the liver shows a focal hypoechoic mass. (*B*) A CEUS image in the same plane at the peak of arterial-phase enhancement shows the mass is enhanced and mildly heterogeneous, appearing slightly less enhanced than the liver. (*C*) A portal venous–phase image shows the mass is now black and washed out relative to the enhanced liver, indicative of a malignant lesion. Enhancement and rapid washout is classic for a metastasis. Three other tiny areas of washout indicate further lesions, occult on baseline.

is performed with low mechanical index to preserve the bubble population while using a subtraction technique that removes the image of the background tissue, allowing visualization of the bubble image only. The timing of imaging for CEUS is similar to that for CT and MR imaging scan but performed with real-time observation to the peak of enhancement in the arterial phase. Intermittent scanning is generally used for observation during the portal and later phases. Because of the noninvasive nature and ease of performance of CEUS, studies may be repeated as required.

THE ONCOLOGY POPULATION

The oncology population is susceptible to the development of a variety of tumor masses. Furthermore, their imaging may be complicated by the presence of preexisting benign pathology. Today, in an era of noninvasive diagnosis and noninvasive treatment options, the detection and characterization of these tumors falls largely within the realm of diagnostic imaging. Furthermore, invasive surgical procedures have been replaced in many instances by image-guided percutaneous procedures, including ablation of tumors by either intense heating (radiofrequency ablation and microwave therapy) or freezing (cryoablation). Because of its resolution and lack of ionizing radiation, US has become the major modality worldwide for the guidance of biopsy and therapeutic techniques. The addition of CEUS at the time of these procedures is now routine for many oncologic patients.

Critical to accurate interpretation of CEUS in oncologic patients are several fundamental observations that allow for accurate prediction of

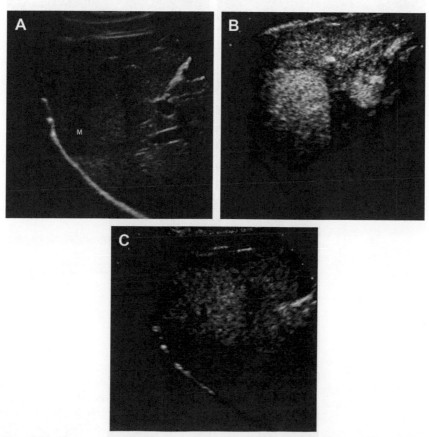

Fig. 2. The value of showing sustained enhancement. A 26-year-old asymptomatic woman with an incidentally discovered liver mass. (*A*) A long-axis view of the liver shows a rather subtle large liver mass (M). (*B*) A CEUS image at the peak of arterial-phase enhancement shows the mass is hypervascular because it appears brighter than the adjacent liver. (*C*) At 4 minutes, the mass is still enhanced greater than the liver and there is a small central non-enhancing scar. Sustained enhancement is typically seen in benign lesions. This is a classic appearance for focal nodular hyperplasia.

malignant disease and provide discriminatory information regarding the specific diagnosis. First, and most important, early investigators became aware that a decline of enhancement of a mass relative to the liver enhancement over time had an association with malignancy.[7] Washout, a term used to describe this decline in enhancement over time, shows less enhancement of a mass relative to the liver and is highly associated with malignant outcome (**Fig. 1**). Furthermore, timing of this washout is discriminatory of cell type of origin in that metastatic disease and cholangiocarcinoma have rapid washout, in less than 1 minute, often beginning as early as 20 seconds.[8] The

washout for nonhepatocellular tumors is also complete such that the tumors appear very black over time relative to the enhanced parenchyma. Hepatocellular carcinoma (HCC), by comparison, shows variable washout intervals but is most often associated with very late and weak washout, not occurring in some patients until close to 5 minutes after contrast agent injection.[9,10] This mandates a long observation period, up to at least 5 minutes, to avoid missing this washout observation.

Most benign masses, by comparison, have a strong tendency for sustained enhancement whereby the mass is equivalent in intensity to or greater than the liver over time (**Fig. 2**).

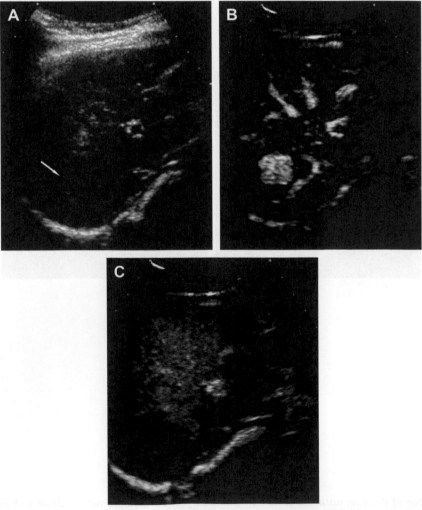

Fig. 3. Classic HCC detected on surveillance US. (*A*) A baseline US image shows a small hypoechoic mass (*arrow*) in the right lobe of a small cirrhotic liver. (*B*) A CEUS image at the peak of arterial-phase enhancement shows classic hypervascularity. (*C*) A CEUS image in the portal venous–phase at 2 minutes. The lesion has washed out relative to the more enhanced liver. (*From* Wilson SR, Burns PN. State of the art microbubble-enhanced US in body imaging: what role? Radiology 2010;257(1):32; with permission.)

A summation of established oncologic applications for CEUS according to the organ studied is presented.

THE LIVER

Liver tumors are the most common indication for abdominal tumor imaging because this large organ is commonly involved in both primary and metastatic disease.

HCC is the third leading cause of cancer deaths in the world. It occurs almost exclusively in those with liver cirrhosis, and known associations include antecedent viral infection with hepatititis B or C, alcoholic cirrhosis, and an increasing association with nonalcoholic fatty liver disease. Therefore, it is now recognized that screening programs in high-risk patients, with US performed every 6 months, provides advantages of early detection, at a time when tumors may still be treated, and down-staging at the time of diagnosis, with improved prognosis.[11,12] Therefore, protocols for the evaluation of small nodules found at US suggest that a nodule with a threshold diameter (D) of 1 cm should motivate CEUS, CT, or MR imaging scan for characterization.[13] In the author's institution, this is performed with CEUS at the time of identification of a nodule on US screening examination. Although classic HCC may be diagnosed at the time of first detection, in many nodules, definitive development of HCC may take time and short interval surveillance, at 3 months, is appropriate. The management of small nodules found on surveillance US is best handled in a multimodality environment and in the author's institution both CEUS and MR imaging are used for

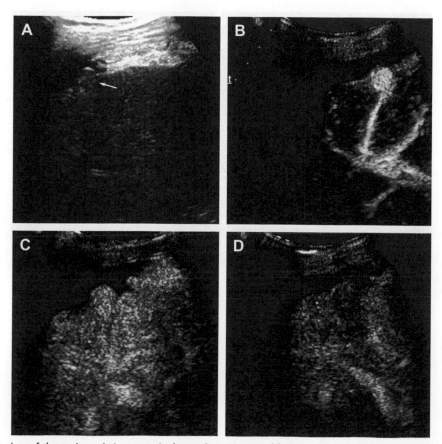

Fig. 4. The value of dynamic real-time scan is shown in a 56-year-old man with hepatitis B virus and a tiny superficial HCC. (*A*) A US image of the right lobe of the liver shows obvious cirrhosis with a suspicious small surface nodule (*arrow*). (*B*) Shows the nodule is hypervascular at the peak of arterial-phase enhancement. (*C*) Shows the nodule is isovascular at 2.75 minutes. It does not show washout. (*D*) Continued observation to 4 minutes shows slow and weak washout, a well-recognized variant of HCC enhancement. (*From* Wilson SR, Burns PN. State of the art microbubble-enhanced US in body imaging: what role? Radiology 2010;257(1):33; with permission.)

routine patient management and follow-up of nodules detected at the time of surveillance (**Fig. 3**).

Tumors develop by a stepwise progression of hepatocarcinogenesis whereby regenerative nodules in the liver evolve into first dysplastic nodules and then small and ultimately larger foci of HCC. This process is accompanied by a progressive decline in the normal arterial and portal flow to the nodule with increasing neoangiogenesis as development of malignant arterial vasculature evolves. This process allows, therefore, for a variety of enhancement patterns, recognition of which improves interpretation of CEUS (**Fig. 4**).

Classic HCC on US shows arterial-phase hypervascularity and washout in the late portal venous phase (**Fig. 5**).[14] Variations of this classic

enhancement pattern include arterial-phase isovascularity or even hypovascularity (**Fig. 6**) and early portal venous–phase washout, which may occur within 1 minute after contrast injection, especially for poorly differentiated tumors. Furthermore, infrequent HCC never washes out. Regenerative nodules, which are typically smaller than 1 cm or 1.5 cm in diameter, show isovascularity of enhancement in both the arterial and portal phases, and dysplastic nodules often show transient hypovascularity followed by sustained isovascularity.

Large HCCs show the same basic enhancement patterns as smaller nodules (**Fig. 7**). The tendency for these tumors to invade the portal veins, however, is classic. These tumor thrombi are characterized by expansion and often

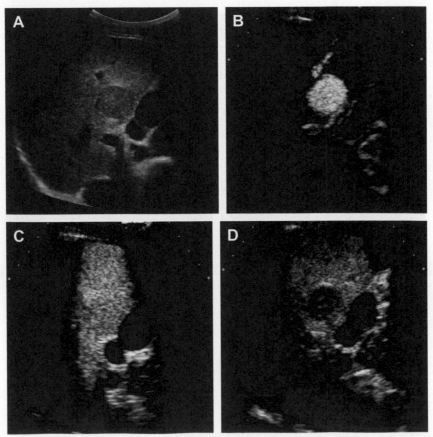

Fig. 5. The value of a long period of observation in the portal venous phase is shown in this 77-year-old man from Hong Kong with a normal liver and serology positive for hepatitis B virus. (*A*) A baseline US image shows a normal liver and a subtle hypoechoic mass. (*B*) A very early arterial-phase image shows the mass is hypervascular even before the liver has begun to enhance. (*C*) At 90 seconds, the mass is invisible because it is isovascular with the liver. (*D*) At 2.5 minutes, the mass shows washout. This delayed washout is classic for HCC and would be missed without a long period of observation.

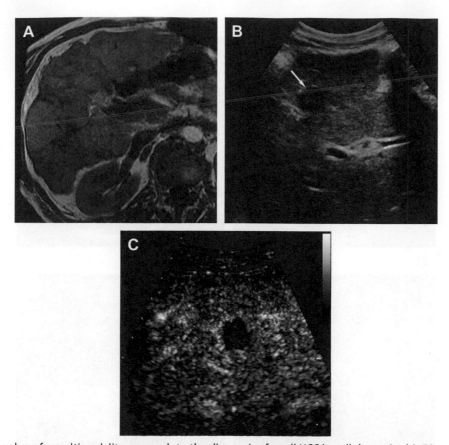

Fig. 6. The value of a multimodality approach to the diagnosis of small HCC is well shown in this 59-year-old man with ethanol and HCV cirrhosis. (*A*) A good quality MR imaging is negative showing no mass on T2-weighted images and no hypervascularity on enhanced scan, representative image shown here. (*B*) A baseline sonogram, shows a single hypoechoic nodule in the right lobe of the cirrhotic liver (*arrow*). (*C*) CEUS arterial-phase image shows clear hypovascularity of the mass. The mass quickly became isovascular and did not show washout. Familiarity with the variations of enhancement patterns of HCC on CEUS prompted request for biopsy, which showed a moderately differentiated HCC. (*From* Wilson SR, Burns PN. State of the art microbubble-enhanced US in body imaging: what role? Radiology 2010;257(1):34; with permission.)

destruction of the vein walls. On CEUS, therefore, tumor thrombi are expansive and often occlusive, showing arterial-phase hypervascularity and portal venous–phase washout, similar to their tumor of origin.

Metastatic disease is characteristic on CEUS, showing rapid washout, generally within 1 minute after injection of contrast and often beginning by as early as 20 seconds (**Fig. 8**).[8] Although the arterial-phase enhancement characteristics are influenced by the blood flow of the primary tumor, the washout remains the same. Therefore, in the arterial phase, these tumors are nonspecific, showing enhancement ranging from diffuse hypervascularity, a rim enhancement pattern of vascularity, isovascularity, and hypovascularity. It is,

therefore, their characteristic rapid washout that allows for their accurate prediction. The improved detection of metastatic disease by sweeping the entire liver during the portal venous phase of enhancement is well documented in that tumors on CEUS show increased conspicuity compared with their appearance on grayscale scan, allowing for detection of more and smaller lesions than on baseline (**Fig. 9**).[15] Lymphomatous involvement of the liver may be diffuse, in which case its detection may be challenging, or it may occur as a tumor mass or masses of variable size. CEUS shows typically arterial-phase enhancement with washout similar to that shown with metastatic disease—that is, rapid and complete washout in less than 1 minute (**Fig. 10**).

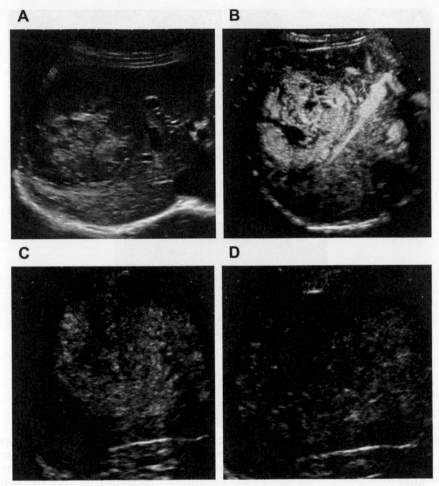

Fig. 7. Large HCC in an 83-year-old woman with no known risk factors for liver cirrhosis. (*A*) A baseline axial US image shows a well-defined heterogeneous mass. (*B*) At the peak of arterial-phase enhancement, the mass is hypervascular and heterogeneous. (*C*) At 2.5 minutes, the mass is still more enhanced than the adjacent liver. (*D*) At 4 minutes, there is washout indicative of malignancy and classic for HCC.

Cholangioarcinoma (CCA) is a rare tumor that arises from the peripheral biliary ducts. Because it may occur in those with normal and cirrhotic livers, its differentiation from both HCC and metastatic disease is essential. On CEUS, its enhancement and washout characteristics resemble metastatic disease, showing arterial-phase enhancement and then rapid washout. Therefore, consideration of CCA is essential in those with a solitary liver tumor and a malignant enhancement pattern characterized by enhancement followed by rapid washout, especially in less than 1 minute. Cholangiocarcinoma on CT and MR imaging scan is described frequently as showing delayed enhancement. This is not shown on CEUS because the delayed enhancement on CT and MR imaging is pseudoenhancement related to

the contrast agent passing into the interstitium of the tumor. CEUS, performed with a purely intravascular bubble, shows true vascular information and does not show this pseudoenhancement.[16,17] Recognition of this potential discordance of CEUS and CECT/CEMR in tumors with this diagnosis is helpful in the multimodality evaluation of small nodules in a cirrhotic liver, contributing to greater accuracy for patient management.

It is this author's belief that CEUS plays a valuable role in the multimodality investigation of nodules in a cirrhotic liver. Whether CEUS has a role as first-line investigation at the same level as CT or MR imaging, however, is inconsistent in national and international guidelines and in practice. CEUS is included in Asian and European guidelines but has recently been removed from

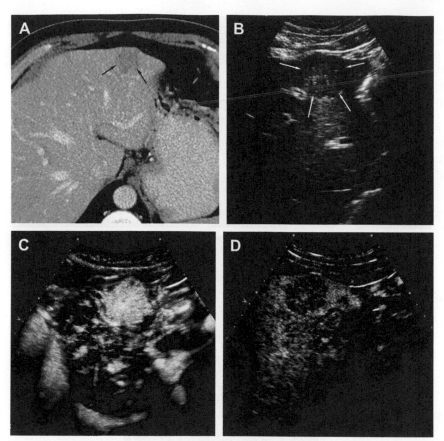

Fig. 8. The value of timing of washout is shown in this 49-year-old man with proved metastasis from colon cancer. (A) An axial CT image shows a low attenuation mass (*arrows*) in the lateral segment of the left lobe. (B) At baseline US, the mass (*arrows*) is slightly exophyptic and of mixed echogenicity. (C) An arterial-phase image from CEUS at the peak of enhancement shows hypervascularity. (D) An image at 45 seconds shows clear washout of the lesion, which had begun at 28 seconds. Rapid washout in less than 1 minute should prompt consideration of metastatic disease or other nonhepatocellular neoplasm.

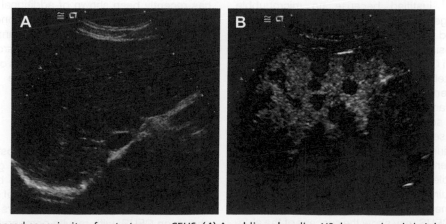

Fig. 9. Increased conspicuity of metastases on CEUS. (A) An oblique baseline US shows only subtle inhomogeneity of the liver. No discrete masses are detected. (B) A portal venous–phase image in the same plane shows multiple black washout areas, classic for metastases.

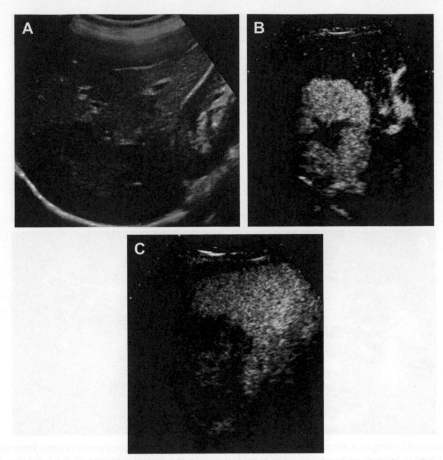

Fig. 10. Lymphoma of the liver, showing as a rather unusual large focal mass. (*A*) A baseline US image shows a large hypoechoic lobulated liver mass. (*B*) It is hypervascular at the peak of arterial-phase enhancement. (*C*) It shows rapid washout, consistent with a nonohepatocellular malignancy.

American guidelines for liver nodule assessment in cirrhosis,[14] justified because no microbubble contrast agent is licensed for the liver in the United States and additionally because of the risk of misdiagnosis of a cholangiocellular carcinoma for HCC when CEUS is used alone (1%–2%). In practice, the likelihood of misdiagnosis is minimal when CEUS is performed by skilled operators.[18] Furthermore, the advantages afforded by the inclusion of CEUS are so varied and extensive as to make its exclusion seemingly impossible.

Monitoring radiofrequency ablation procedures for treatment of HCC and metastatic liver disease is a valuable role for CEUS, allowing for reduction of the requirement for repeat ablation when CEUS is performed at the time of the ablative therapy.[19,20] CEUS may show the success of the ablation and is sensitive for the detection of residual and recurrent tumor (**Fig. 11**).

CEUS of the liver at the time of liver resection has recently been shown of additional benefit to the choice of intraoperative US alone. It is of considerable benefit, altering the planned therapeutic procedure as often as 30% percent of the time by either detection of new lesions or provision of a different diagnosis for those previously known.[21,22]

THE KIDNEY

Renal cell carcinoma (RCC), the most common primary renal tumor, shows variable gross morphology and enhancement on CEUS but shows, in general, enhancement in the arterial phase and then washout over time. Solid tumors are nicely shown on CEUS, with results comparable to their enhancement on CECT or CEMR scan (**Fig. 12**).[23,24] It is, however, cystic RCC where

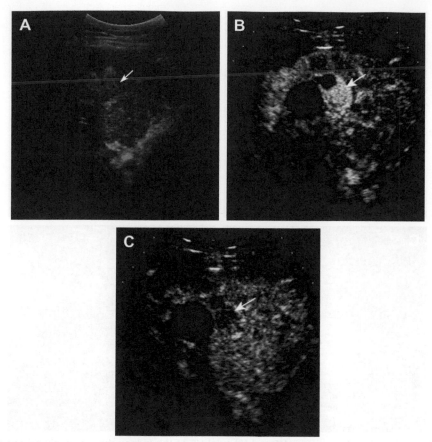

Fig. 11. Value of CEUS for monitoring of RFA. A 63-year-old man with hepatitis B virus cirrhosis and 2 prior RFA treatments for HCC. Surveillance scan. (*A*) A baseline US image shows 2 adjacent echogenic nodules as well as a small hypoechoic nodule (*arrow*). (*B*) At the peak of arterial-phase enhancement, the 2 echogenic nodules are well defined and completely avascular, typical for successfully treated RFA sites. The hypoechoic nodule, however, is now hypervascular (*arrow*). (*C*) At 1.5 minutes, the hypervascular nodule shows washout (*arrow*) indicative of recurrent tumor.

CEUS plays the most highly contributory role (**Fig. 13**). CECT and CEMR are often indeterminate in these tumors whereas US is highly sensitive to the presence of enhancement within mural and septal nodularity. Although less established than its use in the liver, renal CEUS is a rapidly expanding technique, which plays a valuable role for the diagnosis of RCC and for the monitoring of cryotherapy, a popular ablative technique for the treatment of small renal lesions, especially in older patients.

THE PANCREAS

The detection and characterization of pancreatic tumors of variable histology is improved with the addition of CEUS, similar to its use with the liver and kidney (described previously).[25] Pancreatic carcinoma is hypovascular in all phases of enhancement, showing less perfusion of the tumor compared with the adjacent normal parenchyma. Coupled with characteristic grayscale features of a hypoechoic poorly defined mass, frequently obstructing either the pancreatic or the common bile duct, the specificity for diagnosis of this tumor is greatly improved with the additional information of CEUS.

Neuroendocrine tumors characteristically show hypervascularity in the arterial phase and washout at variable rates, depending on their degree of malignancy, with more malignant tumors generally showing more rapid washout.[26] Infrequent metastatic lesions to the pancreas, including from RCC, are indistinguishable from neuroendocrine tumors on the basis of their vascularity (**Fig. 14**).

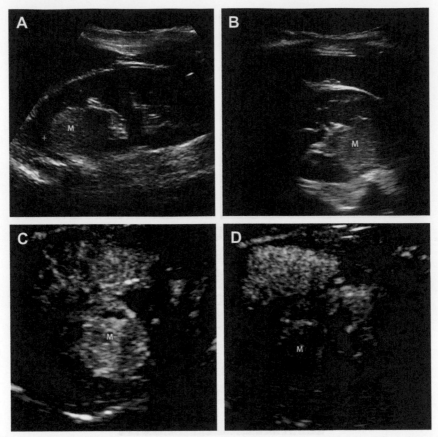

Fig. 12. CEUS of solid RCC. (*A*) Long-axis US and (*B*) axial US of the kidney show a mildly echogenic mass (M). (*C*) At the peak of arterial-phase enhancement, the mass is hypervascular relative to the kidney. (*D*) At 1 minute, there is washout of the mass. CEUS is most often concordant with CT and MR imaging scan for solid renal masses.

THE GALLBLADDER AND BILIARY DUCTS

Tumors within the gallbladder and biliary ducts (**Fig. 15**) are most often malignant if blood flow is confirmed within a solid intraluminal lesion. Although often contributory in the gallbladder to distinguish troublesome sludge balls from tumor, CEUS is most valuable for more confident diagnosis of papillary neoplasms.

OTHER ORGANS AND TUMORS

The author chooses CEUS for the study of any tumor where the addition of blood flow information may be helpful. This includes ovarian and adnexal tumors; gastrointestinal tumors, including carcinoma, carcinoid, and gastrointestinal stromal tumor; and tumors of the prostate. None of these is as established as the liver and kidney applications (described previously).

MONITORING ANGIOGENESIS

A current area of prime interest for CEUS is that of monitoring response of tumors to antiangiogenic therapy. These therapies constitute a new method of tumor treatment that targets the proliferating vasculature of a developing cancer, including drugs specifically designed to inhibit the angiogenic transformation itself.[27] The drugs do not in themselves kill cancer cells, so the tumor often responds without shrinking in size, hence the need for a functional test to determine drug response.[28] Considerable experience accumulated to date suggests that dynamic CEUS, with its advantage of high sensitivity, probability, and a pure intravascular tracer, is a strong candidate for this role.[29–31] Quantitative flow measurement with bubbles is achieved by infusing the agent to a steady level, then using a few high mechanical index pulses to disrupt and clear the image plane

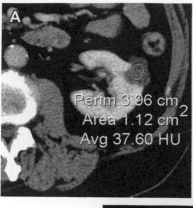
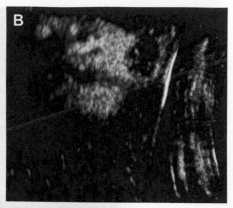
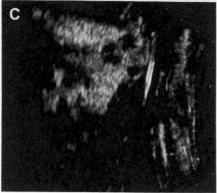

Fig. 13. Value of CEUS in cystic RCC, surgically proved. (*A*) CECT image shows an exophytic left renal mass. It has enhanced 20 HU from the baseline scan (not shown), which is an indeterminate result. Baseline US (not shown) shows a complex cystic and solid renal mass. (*B*) Shows the mass early in the arterial phase of CEUS. The kidney enhances rapidly and appears bright. There are some bubbles within septations of the complex renal mass. (*C*) Shows the mass slightly later and in a slightly different projection with even more enhancement of the mass. CEUS is highly contributory to characterization of cystic RCC, in particular, showing enhancement in cases when CT and MR imaging scan may be indeterminate, as here.

of bubbles after which measurements of its replenishment offers a unique way to quantify microvascular flow and perfusion volume.[32] **Fig. 16** shows an example of a dramatic vascular response of an RCC to a tyrosine receptor kinase inhibitor, with clear reduction in tumor perfusion but no change in tumor volume.

ADVANTAGES OF CEUS

CEUS is a robust and versatile technique that plays a large and contributory role in the management of oncologic patients. For example, a ~equent situation arises when a patient has a por-
' venous–phase CT scan showing small poorly ~ancing masses in the liver. Options include a ~at triphasic CT, an MR imaging scan, or a ~S. In this situation, US with CEUS often shows ~er cysts accounting for the abnormalities or ~how a solid small mass, which may then be

characterized on CEUS as either a malignant or benign insignificant lesion.

The real-time capability of CEUS makes the technique highly sensitive to the documentation of changes in enhancement regardless of their timing or duration. This is invaluable for the study of possible tumor in those at risk for hepatocelluar carcinoma, in particular, where very brief hypervascularity may characterize the tumor in the arterial phase.

CEUS may be repeated as desired and this easily available technique is, therefore, increasingly invaluable in this population.

DISADVANTAGES OF CEUS

No document describing an imaging modality is complete without inclusion of weaknesses of the technique. In general terms, CEUS has the same vulnerabilities as routine sonography, including

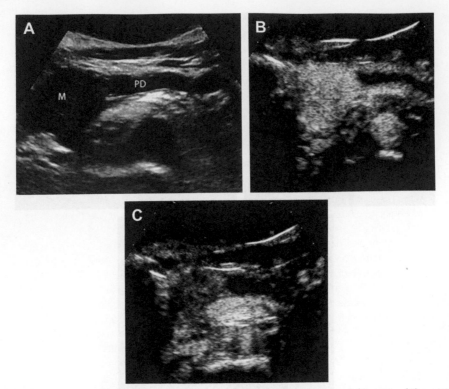

Fig. 14. CEUS improves specificity for diagnosis of pancreatic pathology. (*A*) An axial image of the pancreas shows a dilated pancreatic duct (PD) up to 7 mm with severe pancreatic atrophy. The duct is blocked by a big solid mass (M) in the pancreatic head. (*B*) At the peak of arterial-phase enhancement, the mass is hypervascular. (*C*) At 1 minute, the mass shows washout. These parameters suggest a hypervascular tumor. Biopsy confirms an infrequent metastasis from RCC. Differential diagnosis would include neuroendocrine tumor.

problems relating to patient habitus and ability to cooperate. In terms of liver imaging, the subdiaphragmatic regions may be difficult, and lesions that are small and those that are deep provide further challenge. Commonly, lesions for study of greater than 10-cm depth from the transducer crystal do not show good enhancement. Fat, either in the subcutaneous or peritoneal regions and especially fat deposition in the liver, provides additional severe challenges to the imaging with CEUS.

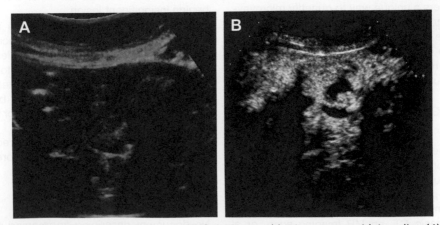

Fig. 15. Biliary papillary cholangiocarcinoma on CEUS. A 78-year-old Asian woman with jaundice. (*A*) An axia age of the CBD shows a dilated duct with a soft tissue mass within the duct. (*B*) A CEUS image in the arterial shows the mass has enhanced. As with all tumors within a cystic structure, CEUS is highly sensitive to the pr of bubbles within the solid components.

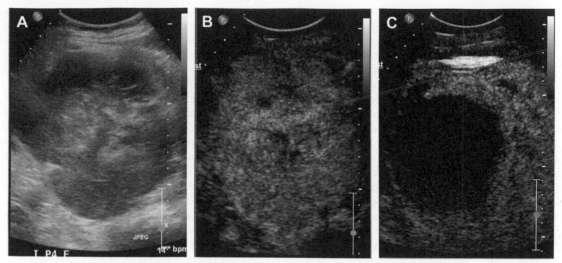

Fig. 16. Monitoring angiogenesis. A 60-year-old woman with RCC. Activity is monitored before and after Sutent, a tyrosine kinase inhibitor. (*A*) A pretreatment US image shows a large tumor in the kidney. There is no normal kidney shown on this image. (*B*) An arterial-phase image from CEUS, in black and white rather than typical chroma, shows the tumor is hypervascular. (*C*) After 14 days of treatment, there is now a large necrotic area within the tumor with reduced vascularity. The mass has changed little in size in spite of the obliteration of the tumor vascularity. (*From* Wilson SR, Burns PN. State of the art microbubble-enhanced US in body imaging: what role? Radiology 2010;257(1):35; with permission.)

SUMMARY

CEUS is a robust and easily performed technique, which may be contributory to management of oncology patients wherever blood flow information may improve interpretation. In this population, CEUS does not challenge for routine metastatic survey but is highly contributory for initial evaluation of those with masses found incidentally or after a purposeful search on US or with other imaging in virtually any organ. CEUS is excellent for tumor follow-up and is especially valuable for resolution of masses indeterminate on either CT or MR imaging scan. It is, therefore, frequently used as a problem solver. In the author's experience, the sensitivity of CEUS to detect tumor vascularity regardless of its timing or duration is indisputable. This plays a critical role in the accurate diagnosis of tumors in many organs. In this era of extreme awareness of the costs of imaging and the risks of ionizing radiation, US with CEUS is undoubtedly a modality of choice.

REFERENCES

1. Cosgrove D, Harvey C. Clinical uses of microbubbles in diagnosis and treatment. Med Biol Eng Comput 2009;47(8):813–26. Available at: http://www.ncbi.nlm.nih.gov/pubmed/19205774. Accessed August 15, 2013.

2. Wilson SR, Burns PN. State of the art microbubble-enhanced US in body imaging: what role? Radiology 2010;257(1):24–39.

3. Albrecht T, Blomley MJ, Burns PN, et al. Improved detection of hepatic metastases with pulse-inversion US during the liver-specific phase of SHU 508A: multicenter study. Radiology 2003;227(2):361–70. Available at: http://www.ncbi.nlm.nih.gov/pubmed/12649417.

4. Dawson P, Cosgrove DO, Grainger RG. Book review. Occup Ther Health Care 1995;9(1):85–6. Available at: http://www.ncbi.nlm.nih.gov/pubmed/23935135.

5. Wilson SR, Kim TK, Jang HJ, et al. Enhancement patterns of focal liver masses: discordance between contrast-enhanced sonography and contrast-enhanced CT and MRI. AJR Am J Roentgenol 2007;189(1):W7–12. Available at: http://www.ncbi.nlm.nih.gov/pubmed/17579140. Accessed August 9, 2013.

6. Piscaglia F, Bolondi L. The safety of sonovue in abdominal applications: retrospective analysis of 23188 investigations. Ultrasound Med Biol 2006;32(9):1369–75. Available at: http://www.ncbi.nlm.nih.gov/pubmed/16965977.

7. Wilson SR, Burns PN. An algorithm for the diagnosis of focal liver masses using microbubble contrast-enhanced pulse-inversion sonography. AJR Am J Roentgenol 2006;186(5):1401–12. Available at: http://www.ncbi.nlm.nih.gov/pubmed/16632737. Accessed August 9, 2013.

8. Murphy-lavallee J, Jang H, Kim TK, et al. Are metastases really hypovascular in the arterial phase? The perspective based on contrast-enhanced ultrasonography. J Ultrasound Med 2007;26(11):1545–56.

9. Fan ZH, Chen MH, Dai Y, et al. Evaluation of primary malignancies of the liver using contrast-enhanced sonography: correlation with pathology. AJR Am J Roentgenol 2006;186(6):1512–9. Available at: http://www.ncbi.nlm.nih.gov/pubmed/16714638. Accessed August 12, 2013.

10. Jang HJ, Kim TK, Burns PN, et al. Enhancement patterns of hepatocellular carcinoma at contrast-enhanced US: comparison with histologic differentiation. Radiology 2007;244(3):898–906.

11. Zhang BH, Yang BH, Tang ZY. Randomized controlled trial of screening for hepatocellular carcinoma. J Cancer Res Clin Oncol 2004;130(7):417–22. Available at: http://www.ncbi.nlm.nih.gov/pubmed/15042359. Accessed August 15, 2013.

12. Takamori R, Wong LL, Dang C, et al. Needle-tract implantation from hepatocellular cancer: is needle biopsy of the liver always necessary? Liver Transpl 2000;6(1):67–72. Available at: http://www.ncbi.nlm.nih.gov/entrez/query.fcgi?cmd=Retrieve&db=PubMed&dopt=Citation&list_uids=10648580.

13. Bruix J, Sherman M. Management of hepatocellular carcinoma. Hepatology 2005;42(5):1208–36. Available at: http://www.ncbi.nlm.nih.gov/pubmed/16250051. Accessed August 8, 2013.

14. Bruix J, Sherman M. Management of hepatocellular carcinoma: an update. Hepatology 2011;53(3):1020–2. Available at: http://www.pubmedcentral.nih.gov/articlerender.fcgi?artid=3084991&tool=pmcentrez&rendertype=abstract.

15. Quaia E, D'Onofrio M, Palumbo A, et al. Comparison of contrast-enhanced ultrasonography versus baseline ultrasound and contrast-enhanced computed tomography in metastatic disease of the liver: diagnostic performance and confidence. Eur Radiol 2006;16(7):1599–609.

16. Burns PN, Wilson SR. Focal liver masses: enhancement patterns on contrast-enhanced images–concordance of US scans with CT scans and MR images. Radiology 2007;242(1):162–74.

17. Chen LD, Xu HX, Xie XY, et al. Intrahepatic cholangiocarcinoma and hepatocellular carcinoma: differential diagnosis with contrast-enhanced ultrasound. Eur Radiol 2010;20(3):743–53. Available at: http://www.ncbi.nlm.nih.gov/pubmed/19760416.

18. Barreiros AP, Piscaglia F, Dietrich CF. Contrast enhanced ultrasound for the diagnosis of hepatocellular carcinoma (HCC): comments on AASLD guidelines. J Hepatol 2012;57(4):930–2. Available at: http://www.ncbi.nlm.nih.gov/pubmed/22739095. Accessed August 12, 2013.

19. Meloni MF, Andreano A, Zimbaro F, et al. Contrast enhanced ultrasound: roles in immediate post-procedural and 24-h evaluation of the effectiveness of thermal ablation of liver tumors. J Ultrasound 2012;15(4):207–14. Available at: http://www.pubmedcentral.nih.gov/articlerender.fcgi?artid=3558080&tool=pmcentrez&rendertype=abstract. Accessed August 15, 2013.

20. Kisaka Y, Hirooka M, Kumagi T, et al. Usefulness of contrast-enhanced ultrasonography with abdominal virtual ultrasonography in assessing therapeutic response in hepatocellular carcinoma treated with radiofrequency ablation. Liver Int 2006;26(10):1241–7.

21. Torzilli G, Del Fabbro D, Palmisano A, et al. Contrast-enhanced intraoperative ultrasonography during hepatectomies for colorectal cancer liver metastases. J Gastrointest Surg 2005;9(8):1148–53 [discussion: 1153–4]. Available at: http://www.ncbi.nlm.nih.gov/pubmed/16269386.

22. Leen E, Ceccotti P, Moug SJ, et al. Potential value of contrast-enhanced intraoperative ultrasonography during partial hepatectomy for metastases: an essential investigation before resection? Ann Surg 2006;243(2):236–40. Available at: http://www.pubmedcentral.nih.gov/articlerender.fcgi?artid=1448920&tool=pmcentrez&rendertype=abstract. Accessed August 15, 2013.

23. Clevert D, Minaifar N, Weckbach S, et al. Multislice computed tomography versus contrast-enhanced ultrasound in evaluation of complex cystic renal masses using the Bosniak classification system. Clin Hemorheol Microcirc 2008;39:171–8.

24. Correas JM, Claudon M, Tranquart F, et al. The kidney: imaging with microbubble contrast agents. Ultrasound Q 2006;22:53–66.

25. D'Onofrio M, Malagò R, Zamboni G, et al. Contrast-enhanced ultrasonography better identifies pancreatic tumor vascularization than helical CT. Pancreatology 2005;5:398–402.

26. D'Onofrio M, Mansueto G, Falconi M, et al. Neuroendocrine pancreatic tumor: value of contrast enhanced ultrasonography. Abdom Imaging 2004;29(2):246–58. Available at: http://www.ncbi.nlm.nih.gov/pubmed/15290954. Accessed August 13, 2013.

27. Kerbel RS, Folkman J. Clinical translation of angiogenesis inhibitors. Nat Rev Cancer 2002;2(10):727–39. Available at: www.ncbi.nlm.nih.gov/pubmed/12360276.

28. Ferrara KW, Merritt CR, Burns PN, et al. Evaluation of tumor angiogenesis with US: imaging, Doppler, and contrast agents. Acad Radiol 2000;7(10):824–39.

29. Goertz DE, Yu JL, Kerbel RS, et al. High-frequency doppler ultrasound monitors the effects of antivascular therapy on tumor blood flow. Cancer R 2002;62:6371–5.

30. Lassau N, Lamuraglia M, Chami L, et Gastrointestinal stromal tumors treated with ima monitoring response with contrast-enh

sonography. AJR Am J Roentgenol 2006;187(5): 1267–73. Available at: http://www.ncbi.nlm.nih.gov/pubmed/17056915. Accessed August 13, 2013.

31. Weskott HP. Emerging roles for contrast-enhanced ultrasound. Clin Hemorheol Microcirc 2008;40:51–71 The Special Contribution of CEUS to Oncology.

32. Arditi M. Second European Symposium on Ultrasound Contrast Imaging Book of Abstracts. Rotterdam (Netherlands): Erasmus Univ; 2004. p. 35.

Endoscopic Ultrasound in Oncology

Vivek Kaul, MD*, Shivangi Kothari, MD

KEYWORDS

- Endoscopic ultrasound • Oncologic imaging • Cancer staging • Fine-needle aspiration • Oncology

KEY POINTS

- Endoscopic ultrasound (EUS) has emerged as an indispensable, dynamic imaging modality in oncology.
- The ability to provide real-time imaging and acquire tissue in a minimally invasive manner is particularly appealing.
- Whereas previously limited to larger centers, EUS is now widely available, even in smaller communities.
- For the vast majority of applications, EUS is a highly accurate, safe, and complementary (to cross-sectional imaging) technology, which has significant impact on the care of patients with cancer.
- Since its inception more than 2 decades ago, EUS technology has made rapid strides in terms of echoendoscope sophistication and processor design and quality.
- In coming years, newer techniques such as elastography and contrast-enhanced EUS will further advance oncologic imaging and continue to benefit patients.

INTRODUCTION

Endoscopic ultrasound (EUS) has emerged as a major technological advance in the realm of endoscopic imaging, particularly in gastrointestinal (GI) oncology. Not only is EUS complementary to cross-sectional imaging (computed tomography [CT], magnetic resonance [MR] imaging) for staging purposes, it also provides a safe, minimally invasive and highly effective portal for accurate tissue diagnosis via fine-needle aspiration (FNA) and core-biopsy techniques.[1]

With ever increasing availability even in smaller centers, EUS has become the standard of care for staging and tissue acquisition in several GI malignancies, including esophageal, gastric, pancreatic, and rectal neoplasms. In addition, EUS has been used for staging and tissue diagnosis of several non-GI tumors (lung, renal, adrenal, and lymphoma).

This article reviews the current role and impact of EUS in oncology along with a review of the recent literature and a brief description of the technical aspects of EUS imaging. EUS in GI oncology is discussed first, followed by a review of non-GI oncologic applications of EUS.

EUS EQUIPMENT

The EUS platform combines the advantages of modern flexible videoendoscopes with those of a high-resolution ultrasound probe/processor, resulting in a powerful dynamic, transluminal imaging modality with real-time tissue-acquisition capabilities. Two types of echoendoscopes are available: the 360° electronic radial echoendoscope (Fig. 1A) with imaging perpendicular to the endoscope axis, and the linear-array echoendoscope (see Fig. 1B) with imaging along the axis of the endoscope and the ability to perform FNA. These

Division of Gastroenterology & Hepatology, Center for Advanced Therapeutic Endoscopy, University of Rochester Medical Center/Strong Memorial Hospital, 601 Elmwood Avenue, Box 646, Rochester, NY 14642, USA
* Corresponding author.
E-mail address: vivek_kaul@urmc.rochester.edu

Ultrasound Clin 9 (2014) 43–52
http://dx.doi.org/10.1016/j.cult.2013.08.004
1556-858X/14/$ – see front matter Published by Elsevier Inc.

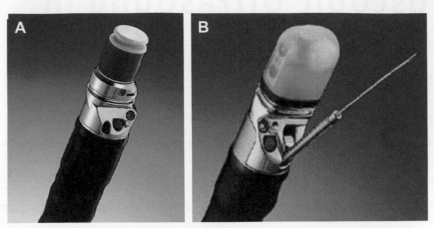

Fig. 1. (*A*) Radial echoendoscope. (*B*) Linear echoendoscope.

endoscopes typically have "oblique viewing" optics, can have a water-filled balloon attached for better acoustic coupling, and can image at frequencies of 5 to 12 MHz, depending on the make and model. Catheter-based "mini-probes" are also available (2–2.6 mm diameter, 20 MHz and 30 MHz); these are mechanical radial ultrasound probes that can be passed into the standard videoendoscope working channel for imaging smaller lesions and those lesions outside the reach of currently available echoendoscopes (eg, imaging in the proximal colon). The newer ultrasound processors combined with the electronic echoendoscopes and ultrasound probes provide high-resolution imaging, especially given the transluminal proximity to the target organs. A wide array of FNA needles is available, ranging from the very thin caliber 25-gauge to the larger 19-gauge "core" needles.

Most EUS procedures can be performed using moderate sedation and on an outpatient basis, with very low overall complication rates.[2,3]

EUS IN GI ONCOLOGY

Esophageal Cancer

EUS has become an integral part of preoperative staging of esophageal cancer. In many aspects, it is complementary to CT and positron emission tomography (PET) imaging, particularly in those patients suspected to have locally advanced disease. Given the survival advantage offered by neoadjuvant therapy, EUS plays an important role in helping identify this subset of patients (ie, those with bulky, locally advanced disease). EUS allows evaluation of the primary tumor (T staging) as well assessment of both regional and distant lymph node status (N staging).[4,5] Invasion of the aorta

and other great vessels, lung, and pleura can also be determined with EUS (**Fig. 2**).

The ability to perform dynamic imaging and obtain tissue in both the mediastinum and abdomen is particularly useful. In the mediastinum, the paraesophageal and para-aortic regions, aorto-pulmonary window, subcarinal space, and inferior mediastinum are easily accessible for examination and tissue sampling. Below the diaphragm, the celiac axis, gastrohepatic ligament, and left lobe of the liver are imaged easily, and the ability to accurately document metastases in these areas has a significant impact on the management of esophageal cancer. EUS has limited utility in patients with established metastatic disease.

For esophageal cancer T staging, typically a radial echoendoscope is used to assess the esophageal-wall layers and depth of infiltration of tumor. The standard criteria used for T staging at EUS are listed in **Table 1**. Bulky and stenotic tumors may not allow passage of echoendoscopes, thus limiting the examination. Many of these patients will require neoadjuvant therapy anyway, given the high probability of locally advanced (T3) and/or nodal disease (N1). Dilation of the stenotic esophageal lumen to 14 to 16 mm may facilitate EUS in these patients; more aggressive dilation is not recommended given the increased risk of perforation, which will then delay cancer management.[6,7] Probe-based and wire-guided sonographic imaging can be performed in this setting, although this is likely of limited benefit from a clinical management perspective. Mediastinal and intra-abdominal lymph nodes can be easily examined and targeted for FNA using the linear-array echoendoscope. The FNA needle path should not cross the primary tumor, to prevent seeding of uninvolved tissue with neoplastic cells.

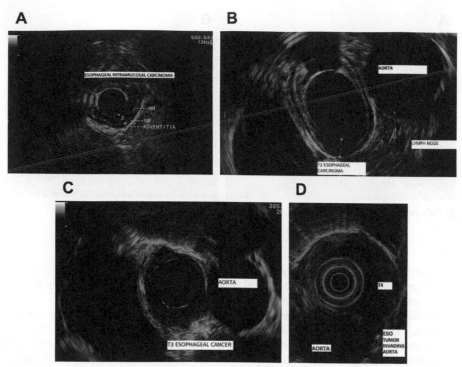

Fig. 2. (*A–D*) Esophageal cancer, EUS staging. MM, muscularis mucosae; SM, submucosa; T, tumor.

EUS has been shown to be highly accurate in the staging of esophageal cancer, particularly for early lesions, when performed by experienced endoscopists. Although some earlier data suggested lower accuracy, a more recent, large meta-analysis reported very high sensitivity, specificity, and accuracy rates.[8,9] An earlier meta-analysis reviewed accuracy of EUS, PET, and CT in the staging of esophageal cancer.[4] For EUS, the sensitivity and specificity for detecting celiac lymph node metastases were 85% and 96%, respectively. Sensitivity and specificity for other regional lymph node metastases were 80% and 70%, respectively. For CT, sensitivity and specificity for regional lymph node metastases were 50% and

83%, respectively. For abdominal lymph node metastases, these values were 42% and 93%, respectively, and for distant metastases 52% and 91%, respectively. For Fluorine-18-fluoro-deoxyglucose PET scanning, sensitivity and specificity for regional lymph node metastases were 57% and 85%, respectively. For distant metastases these values were 71% and 93%, respectively.

Restaging with EUS in patients after neoadjuvant treatment can be difficult, especially in terms of T staging (owing to local inflammation, fibrosis, necrosis, and radiation changes). However, recurrent nodal disease (regional or distant) can be evaluated and targeted for FNA.

Pancreatic Cancer

Pancreatic cancer is the second leading cause of digestive cancer–related death in the United States. Because the vast majority (~85%) of patients will not be candidates for surgical resection at the time of diagnosis, accurate diagnosis and staging is critical to avoid unnecessary surgery in those with unresectable disease. Again, EUS plays a critical complementary role (along with CT) in providing accurate imaging and tissue sampling of pancreatic masses, and has now become the standard tissue-sampling modality for patients found to have a pancreatic mass on CT or MR imaging (**Fig. 3**).

Table 1
EUS T staging for esophageal and other luminal tumors

EUS Imaging	T Stage
Tumor invades into submucosa	T1
Tumor invades into muscularis propria	T2
Tumor invades through muscularis propria	T3
Tumor invades adjacent organs/vessels	T4

A

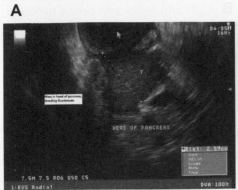

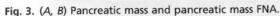

B

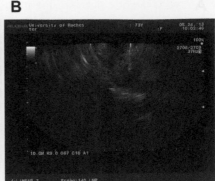

Fig. 3. (*A*, *B*) Pancreatic mass and pancreatic mass FNA.

In a patient with normal (unaltered) foregut anatomy, the entire pancreas can be examined by EUS via the transgastric and transduodenal stations. EUS has a well-established role in the detection, tissue diagnosis, and staging of pancreatic neoplasia. It is particularly good for identifying small (<2 cm) lesions in the pancreas and for obtaining accurate cytologic information with FNA. One of the limitations of EUS in the pancreas is the difficulty in distinguishing an inflammatory (acute or chronic) mass from a neoplastic lesion, on imaging alone; FNA may help clarify the issue in some cases.

The reported accuracy of EUS for T staging of pancreatic cancer is highly variable, ranging from 63% to 94%, with reported accuracies for N staging ranging from 44% to 82%.[10,11] Comparing studies for T staging is difficult because of changes in T-staging criteria over time. Two of the more recent studies showed an accuracy of 63% and 67% for T staging and 67% and 44% for N staging.[12,13] EUS-guided FNA (EUS-FNA) has been reported to have high sensitivity and specificity in diagnosing pancreatic cancer (80%–90% and 100%, respectively).[14,15] The overall complication rates are very low, and the procedure is usually performed on an outpatient basis.

EUS-FNA has been found to be valuable in diagnosing pancreatic cancer when other imaging and tissue-sampling modalities (CT-guided percutaneous biopsy, tissue sampling based on endoscopic retrograde cholangiopancreatography) have been inconclusive or negative. EUS-FNA may aid in the diagnosis and staging of pancreatic cancer in multiple ways:

- Help identify and sample lesions that are too small to be characterized by CT or MR imaging

- Sample lesions that are too encased by surrounding vascular structures to permit safe percutaneous biopsy
- Demonstrate malignant invasion of lymph nodes located in the celiac, para-aortic, retroduodenal, or superior mesenteric regions
- Sample suspected small metastases in the left lobe of the liver
- Confirm peritoneal carcinomatosis via sampling of ascitic fluid

In terms of vascular staging, earlier data suggested that EUS was superior to CT in terms of determining resectability. However, subsequent studies reported lower rates of sensitivity and specificity for vascular invasion as determined by EUS (portal imaging better than mesenteric arterial imaging).[16] The current standard of care for evaluation of a pancreatic mass involves obtaining a contrast-enhanced "pancreatic-protocol" CT scan and, in most cases, an EUS-FNA for confirmation of tissue diagnosis. CT provides excellent vascular staging information and assesses for distant/metastatic tumor, while EUS enables efficient, minimally invasive, highly accurate tissue sampling, and an additional perspective on vascular involvement. If the CT scan suggests distant metastatic disease (confirmed with percutaneous tissue sampling), EUS is typically not performed.

EUS has been found to be particularly useful in patients with suspected pancreatic neuroendocrine tumors (NET), with very high rates of sensitivity, specificity, and accuracy. The ability to localize pancreatic NET when prior imaging was "negative" and the ability to aspirate lesions as small as 5 mm have made EUS-FNA an invaluable tool in this arena.[17]

Overall, EUS is an extremely efficient modality pancreatic tumor imaging and tissue sampli and is complementary to high-quality CT in terms of the preoperative evaluation of the patient with suspected pancreatic neoplasia.

Rectal Cancer

Accurate staging of rectal cancer is important, because management and prognosis are linked to the stage of tumor. Patients with early rectal cancer (stages I and II) may proceed directly to surgery, whereas locally advanced lesions predicate neoadjuvant therapy first, followed by surgery. EUS has been found to have high accuracy for T and N staging in rectal cancer, and to be even superior to CT imaging for T-stage evaluation. A meta-analysis of 90 articles published between 1985 and 2002[18] comparing the staging accuracy of MR imaging, EUS, and CT using pathologic staging as the gold standard, suggested the following:

- For determining muscularis propria invasion (ie, T1 vs T2) EUS and MR imaging had similar sensitivity; specificity of EUS was significantly higher (86% vs 69%).
- For perirectal tissue invasion (T3 disease), the sensitivity of EUS was significantly higher than either MR imaging or CT (90% vs 82% and 79%, respectively).
- For invasion of adjacent organs (T4 disease) and lymph node involvement, estimates for EUS, CT, and MR imaging were comparable.

EUS and MR imaging have been found to have comparable accuracy for T staging, although one study suggested that EUS was more accurate. In terms of N staging, EUS, CT, and MR imaging seem to have similar accuracies as reported in the literature.[19–21]

In general, EUS and MR imaging (with or without an endorectal coil) can both be used for primary tumor staging. MR imaging offers some advantages over EUS: it permits a larger field of view and can visualize more proximal tumors. MRI

tends to be less operator and technique dependent and it allows the study of stenotic tumors.

In terms of restaging after neoadjuvant therapy for rectal cancer, the role for EUS is limited because of local inflammation, radiation changes, and necrosis. Perirectal (extraluminal) tumor recurrence can still be identified and sampled with EUS FNA with high accuracy.

Gastric Cancer

EUS remains a valuable tool in the locoregional staging of gastric carcinoma (**Fig. 4**). Most tumor locations are easily accessed with the dedicated echoendoscope. Lesions high in the gastric fundus may present a technical challenge, especially if they are small, given the limited retroflexion capability of these echoendoscopes and the imaging artifacts created with a nonlinear endoscope position.

Apart from T staging of the primary tumor, EUS allows for tissue sampling of perigastric (including celiac) lymph nodes, evaluation of any liver lesions, and assessment of mediastinal and retroperitoneal/periportal lymph node stations for metastases.

The role of EUS in the staging of gastric cancer has been well studied. One meta-analysis suggested that T staging was superior to N staging when using EUS in gastric cancer. Another meta-analysis concluded that EUS was more accurate for T staging of advanced disease (T3/T4) than for staging of early cancer (T1/T2).[22,23] As in the esophagus, early (superficial) gastric tumors are now increasingly being removed and pathologically staged by endoscopic resection techniques (endoscopic mucosal resection [EMR] and endoscopic submucosal dissection [ESD]). EUS plays a critical role in helping determine which lesions are best suited for these EMR and ESD type interventions. For example, if the muscularis propria is involved by tumor at EUS, endoscopic resection should not be attempted. Equally importantly, if

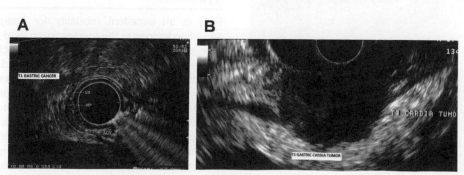

Fig. 4. (A, B) Gastric cancer, EUS staging. ADV, adventitia; MP, muscularis propria; SM, submucosa; T, tumor.

real-time FNA sampling of a lymph node is positive for malignancy during a staging EUS, endoscopic resection should not be contemplated, regardless of T stage.

Liver Masses and Hepatocellular Carcinoma

Hepatocellular carcinoma (HCC) is the sixth most common cancer in the world, with an estimated incidence of more than 650,000 cases per year. Traditionally, transabdominal ultrasonography, CT, and MR imaging have been used for the screening, surveillance, and diagnosis of HCC. However, for some time now there has been interest in evaluating liver lesions by EUS because of the close proximity of the liver to the foregut (stomach and duodenum) (**Fig. 5**). Nguyen and colleagues[24] used EUS-FNA to detect and sample liver lesions in 14 patients suspected to have GI malignancy, including 11 patients in whom lesions were not seen at CT, thereby influencing patient management by more accurate staging of the primary malignancy. In another study, Crowe and colleagues[25] demonstrated similar yield and efficacy for CT-guided FNA and EUS-FNA of liver lesions. Another study by Singh and colleagues[26] found a diagnostic accuracy of 98% with EUS versus 92% with CT for the detection of liver metastases in 132 patients. The study revealed that EUS found a higher number of liver lesions and was able to more accurately characterize very small lesions compared to CT scan.

By contrast, Dodd and colleagues[27] found relatively low sensitivity (58%) of EUS for detection of HCC in a series of 34 patients. A more recent, prospective study compared the accuracy of EUS with that of CT for the detection of primary liver tumors in 17 high-risk patients with abnormal imaging and increased α-fetoprotein levels.[28] The reported diagnostic accuracy of transabdominal ultrasonography, CT, MR imaging, and EUS-FNA was 38%, 69%, 92%, and 94%, respectively.

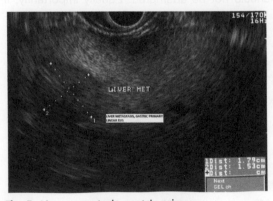

Fig. 5. Liver metastasis, gastric primary.

Current experience suggests that the diagnosis of HCC is highly dependent on the size of the lesion, with tumors smaller than 2 cm being difficult to image and even more difficult to biopsy, especially if the lesion is deep in the liver or in the right lobe. The current evidence suggests that EUS-FNA is a feasible and safe modality for imaging and sampling HCC and liver lesions; however, larger studies and more experience is needed to define its role in this realm.[29]

Subepithelial Lesions in the Gastrointestinal Tract

Both incidentally found and symptomatic (bleeding, obstruction, pain) subepithelial lesions in the gastrointestinal tract can be easily imaged with either dedicated echoendoscopes (radial or linear) or ultrasound mini-probes, the choice of instrument usually being dictated by lesion size and location.[30] FNA can be performed when the examination is performed using a linear echoendoscope. Because of the submucosal/intramural location of these lesions, standard endoscopic forceps (mucosal) biopsies are typically nondiagnostic; hence, these patients are commonly referred for EUS examination.

Gastrointestinal stromal tumors, carcinoids, leiomyomas, and lipomas constitute the vast majority of such lesions referred for EUS evaluation (**Fig. 6**). While real-time EUS imaging helps determine the layer of origin of the lesion, FNA cytology and immunohistochemical staining (eg, chromogranin, CD-117) can help confirm the precise diagnosis and guide management. In the case of larger lesions, fine needle core biopsy samples can also be obtained during real-time EUS, which provide tissue architecture detail and more confidence in the diagnosis. The EUS characteristics of the various subepithelial lesions are shown in **Table 2**.

EUS IN NON-GI ONCOLOGY APPLICATIONS
Lung Cancer and Mediastinal Adenopathy (Lymphoma)

EUS is an excellent modality for imaging and sampling lesions in the mediastinum, and complements cross-sectional imaging and bronchoscopy in the staging of lung cancer.[31,32] In addition to transbronchial biopsy, PET/CT, and mediastinoscopy, EUS has emerged as an additional minimally invasive procedure in staging protocols for lung cancer (**Fig. 7**). With EUS, the aortopulmonary window, subcarinal space, posterior and inferior mediastinum, and paraesophageal lymph node stations can be imaged and sampled fairly easily. In addition, lymphadenopathy below the

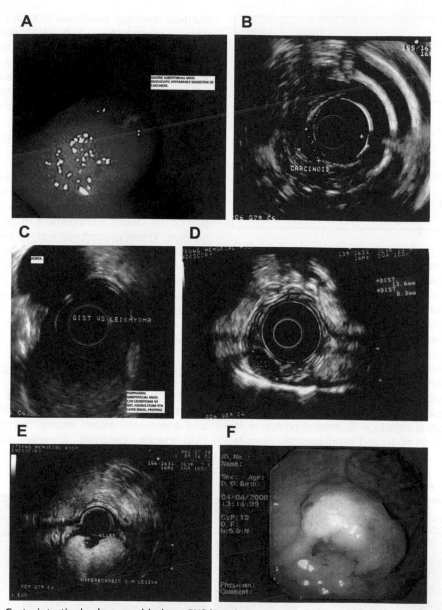

Fig. 6. (*A–F*) Gastrointestinal submucosal lesions, EUS imaging.

diaphragm and a significant portion of the liver can be evaluated also. In one study, EUS, PET, and CT were compared in assessing mediastinal adenopathy in patients with established lung cancer.[33] EUS-FNA was found to be highly sensitive (94%) and specific (100%) for predicting lymph node stage. EUS is also able to directly image and sample lung masses that are in close proximity to and/or in contiguity with the esophageal wall, without significant risk of complications. The ability of EUS to image and sample the adrenal gland for metastatic disease is particularly useful in patients with lung cancer, thereby significantly influencing management.[34]

In patients with suspected lymphoma or mediastinal adenopathy of unexplained etiology, EUS can provide effective diagnostic tissue sampling via FNA, core biopsy, and material for flow cytometry.[35]

Renal Masses

Renal masses and tumors have traditionally been imaged and sampled via a CT-guided approach. EUS is able to easily image both the left kidney (transgastric approach) and the right kidney (transduodenal approach), and has been recently used to assess renal lesions. A small multicenter case

Table 2
EUS features of submucosal lesions in the GI tract

Lesion	EUS Features	Layer of Origin/ Location
Lipoma	Hyperechoic	Submucosa
Leiomyoma	Hypoechoic, discrete	Muscularis mucosae Muscularis propria
GI stromal tumor	Hypoechoic, discrete	Muscularis propria
Carcinoid	Hypoechoic, discrete	Submucosa

series has demonstrated the feasibility and safety of EUS-FNA for kidney lesions. In the series by De Witt and colleagues,[36] 15 patients with kidney masses (median diameter 32 mm; range 11–60 mm) located in the upper (n = 12) and lower (n = 3) poles of the left (n = 10) and right (n = 5) kidneys, respectively, underwent EUS-FNA. Initial mass detection was by previous imaging in 13 (87%) patients or by EUS in 2 (13%) patients. Results of EUS-FNA were diagnostic of (n = 7) or highly suspicious for (n = 1) renal cell carcinoma (RCC), atypical cells (n = 2), oncocytoma (n = 1), benign cyst (n = 1), and nondiagnostic (n = 1).

Surgical resection confirmed RCC in 7 patients in whom preoperative EUS-FNA demonstrated RCC (n = 5) or oncocytoma (n = 1), or was not performed (n = 1). No complications were reported in this study. Although these results are encouraging, more studies are needed to further assess the role of EUS in the realm of renal mass evaluation.

EUS-BASED THERAPEUTIC INTERVENTIONS IN ONCOLOGY

In addition to the imaging and tissue-acquisition capabilities, there are several specific EUS-based interventions that can be performed as part of the overall management of certain malignancies. These procedures include celiac plexus neurolysis, EUS-guided biliary access, fiducial placement for more targeted radiotherapy, and injection of chemotherapeutic agents into tumor.[37] A detailed discussion of these interventions is undertaken in the article Therapeutic Applications of Endoscopic Ultrasound by Kothari and Kaul elsewhere in this issue.

COMPLICATIONS OF EUS AND EUS-FNA

Apart from the usual complications associated with endoscopy (cardiovascular events, sedation- and anesthesia-related issues), some additional EUS-specific potential adverse events merit

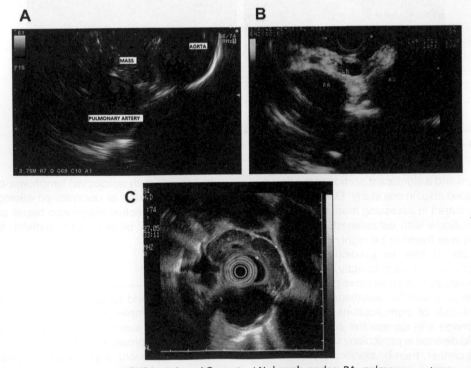

Fig. 7. (A–C) Mediastinal lesions, EUS imaging. AO, aorta; LN, lymph nodes; PA, pulmonary artery.

discussion. These events are primarily related to the design and functionality of echoendoscopes (long rigid tip, oblique viewing optics) and the nature of transluminal interventions (FNA, fine-needle biopsy) typically performed during EUS. The risk for GI perforation and bleeding in a prospective study of 300 patients was 0% to 0.4%.[3,38] The bleeding rate was reported to be up to 6% in one study of FNA in pancreatic cystic lesions.[39] Infectious complications have been reported in 0.3% of EUS-FNA procedures. Infection has been reported with FNA of cysts, in both the mediastinum and the abdomen; the risk is markedly decreased with use of prophylactic antibiotics. Pancreatitis after FNA of solid and cystic lesions has been reported at rates of 0.6% and 2%, respectively.[40] Although usually mild, severe pancreatitis has also been reported. Avoidance of normal pancreatic tissue and limiting the number of needle passes may help mitigate this risk.

SUMMARY

EUS has emerged as an indispensable, dynamic imaging modality in oncology. The ability to provide real-time imaging and acquire tissue in a minimally invasive manner is particularly appealing. Whereas previously limited to larger centers, EUS is now widely available, even in smaller communities.

For the vast majority of applications, EUS is a highly accurate, safe, and complementary (to cross-sectional imaging) technology that has significant potential in terms of influencing the care of patients with cancer. Since its inception more than 2 decades ago, EUS technology has made rapid strides in terms of echoendoscope sophistication, and processor design and quality. In the coming years, newer techniques such as elastography and contrast-enhanced EUS will further advance oncologic imaging and continue to benefit patients with cancer.

REFERENCES

1. Varadarajulu S, Fockens P, Hawes RH. Best practices in endoscopic ultrasound-guided fine-needle aspiration. Clin Gastroenterol Hepatol 2012;10(7): 697–703.
2. Eloubeidi MA, Tamhane A, Varadarajulu S, et al. Frequency of major complications after EUS-guided FNA of solid pancreatic masses: a prospective evaluation. Gastrointest Endosc 2006;63(4):622–9.
3. O'Toole D, Palazzo L, Arotçarena R, et al. Assessment of complications of EUS-guided fine-needle aspiration. Gastrointest Endosc 2001;53(4):470–4.
4. van Vliet EP, Heijenbrok-Kal MH, Hunink MG, et al. Staging investigations for oesophageal cancer: a meta-analysis. Br J Cancer 2008;98(3):547–57.
5. Thosani N, Singh H, Kapadia A, et al. Diagnostic accuracy of EUS in differentiating mucosal versus submucosal invasion of superficial esophageal cancers: a systematic review and meta-analysis. Gastrointest Endosc 2012;75(2):242–53.
6. Pfau PR, Ginsberg GG, Lew RJ, et al. Esophageal dilation for endosonographic evaluation of malignant esophageal strictures is safe and effective. Am J Gastroenterol 2000;95(10):2813–5.
7. Wallace MB, Hawes RH, Sahai AV, et al. Dilation of malignant esophageal stenosis to allow EUS guided fine-needle aspiration: safety and effect on patient management. Gastrointest Endosc 2000;51(3): 309–13.
8. Young PE, Gentry AB, Acosta RD, et al. Endoscopic ultrasound does not accurately stage early carcinoma or high grade dysplasia of the esophagus. Clin Gastroenterol Hepatol 2010;8(12):1037.
9. Puli SR, Reddy JB, Bechtold ML, et al. Staging accuracy of esophageal cancer by endoscopic ultrasound: a meta-analysis and systematic review. World J Gastroenterol 2008;14(10):1479–90.
10. Săftoiu A, Vilmann P. Role of endoscopic ultrasound in the diagnosis and staging of pancreatic cancer. J Clin Ultrasound 2009;37(1):1.
11. De Witt J, Devereaux BM, Lehman GA, et al. Comparison of endoscopic ultrasound and computed tomography for the preoperative evaluation of pancreatic cancer: a systematic review. Clin Gastroenterol Hepatol 2006;4(6):717.
12. Soriano A, Castells A, Ayuso C, et al. Preoperative staging and tumor resectability assessment of pancreatic cancer: prospective study comparing endoscopic ultrasonography, helical computed tomography, magnetic resonance imaging, and angiography. Am J Gastroenterol 2004;99(3):492.
13. De Witt J, Devereaux B, Chriswell M, et al. Comparison of endoscopic ultrasonography and multidetector computed tomography for detecting and staging pancreatic cancer. Ann Intern Med 2004;141(10): 753.
14. Raut CP, Grau AM, Staerkel GA, et al. Diagnostic accuracy of endoscopic ultrasound-guided fine-needle aspiration in patients with presumed pancreatic cancer. J Gastrointest Surg 2003;7(1):118–26.
15. Shin HJ, Lahoti S, Sneige N. Endoscopic ultrasound-guided fine-needle aspiration in 179 cases: the M. D. Anderson Cancer Center experience. Cancer 2002;96(3):174–80.
16. Ahmad NA, Lewis JD, Ginsberg GG. EUS in preoperative staging of pancreatic cancer. Gastrointest Endosc 2000;52(4):463.
17. Anderson MA, Carpenter S, Thompson NW, et al. Endoscopic ultrasound is highly accurate and

directs management in patients with neuroendo-crine tumors of the pancreas. Am J Gastroenterol 2000;95(9):2271–7.

18. Bipat S, Glas AS, Slors FJ, et al. Rectal cancer: local staging and assessment of lymph node involvement with endoluminal US, CT, and MR imaging—a meta-analysis. Radiology 2004;232(3):773–83.

19. Guinet C, Buy JN, Ghossain MA, et al. Comparison of magnetic resonance imaging and computed to-mography in the preoperative staging of rectal can-cer. Arch Surg 1990;125(3):385.

20. Rifkin MD, Ehrlich SM, Marks G. Staging of rectal carcinoma: prospective comparison of endorectal US and CT. Radiology 1989;170(2):319.

21. Puli SR, Reddy JB, Bechtold ML. Accuracy of endo-scopic ultrasound to diagnose nodal invasion by rectal cancers: a meta-analysis and systematic re-view. Ann Surg Oncol 2009;16(5):1255.

22. Puli SR, Batapati Krishna Reddy J, Bechtold ML, et al. How good is endoscopic ultrasound for TNM staging of gastric cancers? A meta-analysis and systematic review. World J Gastroenterol 2008; 14(25):4011–9.

23. Mocellin S, Marchet A, Nitti D. EUS for the staging of gastric cancer: a meta-analysis. Gastrointest En-dosc 2011;73(6):1122–34.

24. Nguyen P, Feng JC, Chang KJ. Endoscopic ultra-sound (EUS) and EUS-guided fine-needle aspiration (FNA) of liver lesions. Gastrointest Endosc 1999; 50(3):357–61.

25. Crowe DR, Eloubeidi MA, Chhieng DC, et al. Fine-needle aspiration biopsy of hepatic lesions: computerized tomographic-guided versus endo-scopic ultrasound-guided FNA. Cancer 2006; 108(3):180–5.

26. Singh P, Mukhopadhyay P, Bhatt B, et al. Endo-scopic ultrasound versus CT scan for detection of the metastases to the liver: results of a prospective comparative study. J Clin Gastroenterol 2009;43(4): 367–73.

27. Dodd GD 3rd, Miller WJ, Baron RL, et al. Detection of malignant tumors in end-stage cirrhotic livers: ef-ficacy of sonography as a screening technique. Am J Roentgenol 1992;159(4):727–33.

28. Singh P, Erickson RA, Mukhopadhyay P, et al. EUS for detection of the hepatocellular carcinoma: results of a prospective study. Gastrointest Endosc 2007; 66(2):265–73.

29. Maheshwari A, Kantsevoy S, Jagannath S, et al. Endoscopic ultrasound and fine-needle aspiration for the diagnosis of hepatocellular carcinoma. Clin Liver Dis 2010;14(2):325–32.

30. Parmar K, Waxman I. Endosonography of submuco-sal lesions. Tech Gastrointest Endosc 2000;2:89–93.

31. Vázquez-Sequeiros E, González-Panizo-Tamargo F, Barturen A, et al. The role of endoscopic ultrasound guided fine needle aspiration (EUS-FNA) in non small cell lung cancer (NSCLC) patients: SEED-SEPD-AEG Joint Guideline. Rev Esp Enferm Dig 2013;105(4):215–24.

32. Ogita S, Robbins DH, Blum RH, et al. Endoscopic ul-trasound fine-needle aspiration in the staging of non-small-cell lung cancer. Oncology (Williston Park) 2006;20(11):1419–25.

33. Fritscher-Ravens A, Bohuslavizki KH, Brandt L, et al. Mediastinal lymph node involvement in potentially resectable lung cancer: comparison of CT, positron emission tomography, and endoscopic ultrasonog-raphy with and without fine-needle aspiration. Chest 2003;123(2):442–51.

34. Sharma R, Ou S, Ullah A, et al. Endoscopic ultra-sound (EUS)-guided fine needle aspiration (FNA) of the right adrenal gland. Endoscopy 2012; 44(Suppl 2 UCTN):E385–6.

35. Catalano MF, Nayar R, Gress F, et al. EUS-guided fine needle aspiration in mediastinal lymphadenopa-thy of unknown etiology. Gastrointest Endosc 2002; 55(7):863–9.

36. DeWitt J, Gress FG, Levy MJ, et al. EUS-guided FNA aspiration of kidney masses: a multicenter U.S. experience. Gastrointest Endosc 2009;70(3):573–8.

37. Kaul V, Adler DG, Conway JD, et al. Interventional EUS. Gastrointest Endosc 2010;72(1):1–4.

38. Wang KX, Ben QW, Jin ZD, et al. Assessment of morbidity and mortality associated with EUS-guided FNA: a systematic review. Gastrointest Endosc 2011;73(2):283–90.

39. Varadarajulu S, Eloubeidi MA. Frequency and signif-icance of acute intracystic hemorrhage during EUS-FNA of cystic lesions of the pancreas. Gastrointest Endosc 2004;60(4):631–5.

40. Eloubeidi MA, Gress FG, Savides TJ, et al. Acute pancreatitis after EUS-guided FNA of solid pancre-atic masses: a pooled analysis from EUS centers in the United States. Gastrointest Endosc 2004; 60(3):385–9.

Therapeutic Applications of Endoscopic Ultrasound

Shivangi Kothari, MD, Vivek Kaul, MD*

KEYWORDS

- Therapeutic • Endoscopic ultrasound • Fine needle injection • Oncology • Fiducial placement
- Celiac plexus neurolysis

KEY POINTS

- Endoscopic ultrasound (EUS) technology has evolved over the last few decades from a diagnostic modality to one that serves as a platform for multiple therapeutic interventions.
- A few EUS-guided therapeutic techniques (eg, anti-tumor agent injection, EUS-guided ablation, and EUS-guided brachytherapy) appear promising in selected patients with cancer.
- Further large prospective randomized trials are needed to evaluate the safety, efficacy, and feasibility of some of these interventions.
- Techniques such as celiac plexus neurolysis for analgesia, EUS-guided endoscopic retrograde cholangiopancreatography for difficult-to-access bile ducts obstructed by tumor or due to difficult anatomy, EUS guided gold fiducial placement to guide radiation therapy and delivery of antitumor agents are just some of the therapeutic applications of EUS in patients with cancer.
- In this dynamic, constantly evolving field of interventional endoscopy, newer minimally invasive therapeutic options for patients with cancer will continue to develop, and several of these will likely be EUS-based interventions.

INTRODUCTION

Endoscopic ultrasound (EUS) has been widely used and is now considered the diagnostic procedure of choice for tissue sampling of pancreatic tumors. It is also used routinely for staging and diagnosis of many gastrointestinal and biliary lesions. EUS-guided fine needle aspiration (FNA) has emerged as a minimally invasive, safe, and accurate technique for tissue sampling. With the development of the linear array EUS echoendoscopes and FNA techniques, various management options have emerged for therapeutic applications of EUS in patients with cancer. Various therapeutic applications of EUS, such as EUS-guided ablation, celiac plexus neurolysis (CPN), EUS-guided brachytherapy and ablation, EUS-guided fiducial marker placement, EUS-guided bile duct access, and delivery of antitumor agents, are discussed in this article.

CPN and Celiac Plexus Block

Intractable abdominal pain is commonly seen in patients with chronic pancreatitis and pancreatic cancer. Celiac plexus block (CPB) and CPN, respectively, have been used to decrease the pain and opiate requirements in such patients. Before the advent of EUS, computed tomography (CT) -guided paraspinal and transabdominal approaches were used but serious complications like paraplegia and pneumothorax were reported. EUS guidance provides better delineation of celiac anatomy and is safe and effective. When compared with CT, EUS provides a more targeted approach, providing better delineation

Financial Disclosure: The authors have no relevant financial disclosures.
Division of Gastroenterology & Hepatology, Center for Advanced Therapeutic Endoscopy, University of Rochester Medical Center/Strong Memorial Hospital, 601 Elmwood Avenue, Box 646, Rochester, NY 14642, USA
* Corresponding author.
E-mail address: vivek_kaul@urmc.rochester.edu

Ultrasound Clin 9 (2014) 53–65
http://dx.doi.org/10.1016/j.cult.2013.08.002
1556-858X/14/$ – see front matter Published by Elsevier Inc.

of the anatomy because of the proximity of the transducer to the celiac plexus and the ability to perform the procedure with real-time imaging.[1] CPN is a chemical splanchnicectomy of the celiac plexus leading to ablation of the pain transmitting afferent nerve fibers from the intra-abdominal viscera. Three techniques of EUS-guided CPN have been reported: traditional or bilateral CPN, broad plexus neurolysis, and celiac ganglion neurolysis (CGN).[1] In the traditional and most commonly used technique for EUS-CPN, using a 19-gauge or 22-gauge needle, a mixture of bupivacaine (0.25%–1%) and ethanol (95%–99%) is injected anterior to the celiac trunk. Sahai and colleagues[2] have demonstrated the efficacy of bilateral injection compared with unilateral CPN with mean pain reduction of 70% versus 46% respectively. In the bilateral EUS-CPN approach, injection is performed on both sides of the celiac trunk as compared to a central single injection with the traditional approach. In broad celiac plexus neurolysis, the entire injection is given anterior and caudal to the superior mesenteric artery.[3] In CGN, direct injection of the ganglion is performed and this has been reported to be highly effective in patients with pancreatic cancer and chronic pancreatitis.[4] **Fig. 1** demonstrates celiac ganglion neurolysis. Suzuki and colleagues[5] reported 94% pain relief in 17 patients undergoing direct ganglia injection.

Celiac plexus block (CPB) involves injection of steroid with an anesthetic agent into the celiac plexus region, whereas CPN involves using a sclerosant agent such as alcohol with an anesthetic agent. Absolute alcohol is reserved for use in patients with unresectable pancreatic cancer because of its effect of inducing fibrosis.[6] In a recent randomized multicenter trial of EUS-CGN versus EUS-CPN in upper abdominal cancer, EUS-CGN was found to be superior to EUS-CPN in pain relief.[7]

In a meta-analysis of 6 studies with a total of 221 patients of EUS-guided CPB in chronic pancreatitis, CPB was effective in alleviating chronic pancreatitis pain in 51.46% of patients. For pancreatic cancer, analysis of 5 relevant studies with a total of 119 patients revealed EUS-CPN to be effective in alleviating pain in 72.54% of patients.[8] Although CPN may not improve survival, it has been associated with improved pain control and reduced narcotic use thereby leading to decreased constipation.[9] Commonly reported complications of CPN have been transient hypotension, diarrhea, increase in abdominal pain, and abscess formation. Three cases of postblock empyema have been reported possibly because of infection tracking into the chest from the celiac plexus.[4,10–12] No major neurologic complications have been reported with CPN. One case of fatality has been reported by Gimeno-Garcia and colleagues[13] after CPN.

Thus CPN and CPB can be considered in carefully selected patients with poorly controlled abdominal pain secondary to pancreatic cancer and chronic pancreatitis, respectively.

EUS-guided Brachytherapy

Advanced pancreatic cancer can be controlled locally with the help of radiation therapy. Some of the radiation therapies include fractional external beam radiation therapy with chemotherapy, interstitial brachytherapy, and image-guided radiotherapy. Interstitial brachytherapy has been used conventionally to control malignancies of the prostate, breast, and brain. Brachytherapy has been considered to have potential therapeutic effect in patients with unresectable pancreatic cancer and in a case of paraaortic lymph node metastasis of pancreatic cancer.[14,15] This technique involves radioactive seeds implanted directly into the tumor followed by local emission of gamma rays, thus leading to tissue

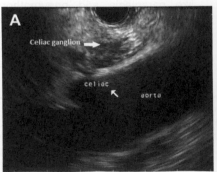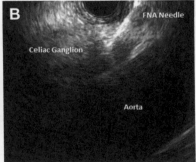

Fig. 1. Celiac ganglion neurolysis. (*A*) The celiac axis ganglion. (*B*) EUS-guided FNI into the celiac ganglion.

destruction. Traditionally, these radiation seeds are placed operatively or using a percutaneous approach. Sun and colleagues[16] in 2005 first reported EUS-guided brachytherapy in a porcine model using 6 pigs. Radioactive iodine 125-seeds were implanted into normal pig pancreas under EUS visualization. Repeat EUS on day 7 demonstrated heterogenous hypoechoic lesions surrounding the seeds in all pigs. On autopsy, it was noted that localized necrosis surrounded by fibrotic tissue with mild inflammation was present around the seeds thus indicating local tissue destruction from the seeds. Sun and colleagues[17] and Jin and colleagues[18] have evaluated EUS-guided placement of radioactive iodine seeds in patients with locally advanced pancreatic cancer. In 2006, Sun and colleagues reported EUS-guided placement of a mean of 22 radioactive seeds per patient in a study of 15 patients. In a median follow-up of 10.6 months, "partial" response was seen in 27% patients, "minimal" response in 20% patients, and "stable" disease in 33% patients. Clinical benefit of pain reduction was seen in 30% of patients. Pancreatitis and pseudocyst formation were seen in 3 patients. Hematologic toxicity was reported in 3 patients. Jin and colleagues reported a study of 22 patients with locally advanced pancreatic cancer. In this study, in addition to the EUS-guided placement of radioactive seeds, all patients received gemcitabine-based 5-Fluorouracil chemotherapy 1 week after the brachytherapy. The median follow-up of these patients was 9.3 months. Partial remission was achieved in 13.6% of patients and the disease remained stable in 45.5% of patients. The pain score initially dropped significantly after the brachytherapy but increased again 1 month later. No obvious complications were reported. Cancer progressed in 20 patients and all patients died over the follow-up period of 2 years. EUS-guided brachytherapy has been reported in patients with primary head and neck cancers[19] and in one case of esophageal cancer metastasizing to celiac lymph node.[20] EUS-guided brachytherapy seems encouraging in the initial animal and clinical studies. Further studies are needed in evaluating the safety and efficacy of this technique in a larger patient population along with the evaluation of the safety of the gastroenterologist handling the radioactive material in the endoscopy suite.

EUS-guided Fiducial Marker Placement

Image-guided radiotherapy platforms include stereotactic body radiation therapy and intensity-modulated radiation therapy. These 2 therapies have been considered less toxic when compared to the conventional external fractionated radiotherapy because of the accuracy and precision of these treatments. Cyberknife frameless radiosurgery system (Accuray, Sunnyvale, CA, USA) involves the use of image-guided radiotherapy. Intracranial lesions are treated using bony landmarks for reference points. In nonintracranial tumors fiducial markers or radiographic implants are used as reference points for delivery of this therapy. Traditionally, placement of fiducial markers has been performed under CT-guided percutaneous approach or by surgery. Pishvaian and colleagues[21] successfully demonstrated the placement of fiducial markers using the EUS route in 6 of 7 patients with pancreatic cancer without any reported complications. The technique in EUS-guided fiducial placement involves the use of linear array echoendoscope. With the help of linear array echoendoscope, the pancreatic tumor is localized. The sterile gold fiducial (0.8 mm diameter × 3–5 mm length) is preloaded at the tip of a 19-gauge FNA needle after slight retraction of the stylet. The tip of the needle is then sealed using bone wax to prevent dislodging the fiducial from the needle tip. The tumor is identified and, after confirming lack of intervening structures, the needle is advanced into the tumor and the stylet is pushed into the needle, deploying the fiducials into the tumor (**Fig. 2**).

Fluoroscopic visualization can be used for confirmation; however, fiducial placement can be performed under EUS visualization alone.[22,23]

Ideal fiducial geometry (IFG), as recommended for image-guided radiation therapy for the use of the Cyberknife system, is described as at least 3 fiducials with a minimum distance of greater than 2 cm, minimum interfiducial angle of more than 15°, and noncollinear placement in the imaging plane.[24] The clinical significance of achieving IFG has not yet been clearly established. In a recent study by Majumder and colleagues,[23] comparing fiducial placement by EUS and surgery to attain IFG, it was reported that IFG was significantly higher by surgical placement. However, fiducial tracking for Cyberknife therapy was successful in 90% patients in the EUS group compared with 82% of patients in the surgery group, thus demonstrating that achieving IFG seemed unnecessary for successfully tracking and delivering radiotherapy.

Postprocedure complication rates with EUS-guided fiducial placement have been low with reports of mild abdominal pain and pancreatitis.[23] Technical success of EUS-guided fiducial placement has been reported in 11 of 13 patients with mediastinal and intra-abdominal malignancy by Pishvaian and colleagues.[21] No major complications related to the placement of the fiducial

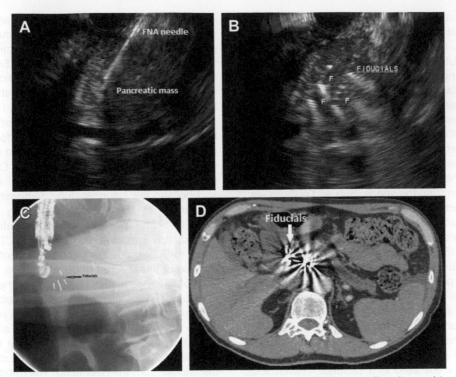

Fig. 2. EUS-guided gold fiducial placement into pancreatic neck tumor. (*A*) FNA needle advanced into the mass. (*B*) Fiducials seen on EUS. (*C*) Fiducials seen on fluoroscopy. (*D*) Fiducials seen on CT.

were noted in the study. It can sometimes be technically challenging to place the fiducial due to the stiffness of the 19-gauge needle, or when using the 5-mm long fiducial, or due to location of the tumor such as in the head of the pancreas. Some of these issues can be overcome by straightening the endoscope, using smaller fiducials, or using a more flexible/smaller gauge needle.

Larger randomized controlled trials are required to compare the benefit of image-guided radiotherapy for pancreatic cancer with conventional external radiotherapy and, in turn, assess the significance of EUS-guided fiducial placement. Larger studies are also needed to evaluate the overall safety of fiducials because migration of fiducials and infections are also some of the concerns.

Ethanol Ablation

With the evolution of EUS and EUS FNA since the 1990s, various therapeutic EUS techniques have also developed including EUS-guided fine needle injection (FNI). Ethanol has been used percutaneously to ablate hepatic cysts, kidney cysts, and liver and adrenal tumors.[25–28] Ethanol causes cell death by breaking down the cell membrane, causing protein denaturation and vascular occlusion. EUS guidance allows real-time imaging and

access to lesions not accessible by the percutaneous route. EUS can also precisely identify lesions in the pancreas and deliver agents to the targeted tissue with real-time imaging, thus reducing damage to nontumor/normal tissue. Safety and feasibility of EUS-guided ethanol ablation in the pancreas in an animal model has been reported.[29] With the advent of sophisticated radiologic imaging studies like CT scan and MR imaging, there is an increased detection of pancreatic cystic neoplasms. Cystic lesions of the pancreas such as intraductal papillary mucinous neoplasms and mucinous cystic neoplasms have malignant potential and these may require surgical resection.

EUS-guided ethanol injection for lavage and ablation of pancreatic cystic lesions was first reported by Gan and colleagues.[30] Twenty-five patients with pancreatic cysts (mucinous cystic neoplasms = 13, intraductal papillary mucinous neoplasms = 4, serous cystadenoma = 3, pseudocyst = 3, uncertain etiology = 2) were treated with different concentrations of ethanol (5%–80%) for 3 to 5 minutes. The cyst was punctured with a 22-gauge needle; the fluid was aspirated, and the cyst was collapsed. Cyst fluid was sent to evaluate for carcinoembryonic antigen (CEA) and amylase levels. Ethanol was then injected into the collapsed cyst and lavaged for 3 t

5 minutes alternating filling and emptying the cyst. No complications were reported in the study and 35% of patients had complete resolution of the cysts. Five patients who underwent surgical resection had histologic evidence of epithelial ablation.

A multicenter, randomized prospective trial comparing the change of pancreatic cyst size after EUS-guided lavage with 80% ethanol or saline solution reported a greater decrease in size of pancreatic cystic tumor in the ethanol injection group. Overall, there was a complete resolution of the pancreatic cystic tumors in 33.3% of patients. Major complications such as abdominal pain, significant bleeding, and acute pancreatitis in the 2 groups were similar.[31]

Oh and colleagues[32] performed EUS-guided ethanol lavage with paclitaxel of pancreatic cysts and found complete resolution of the pancreatic cystic tumors in 11 of 14 patients. The same group later performed a study with 52 patients with a longer follow-up period, reporting complete resolution of the pancreatic cysts in 62% patients using EUS-guided injection and lavage with ethanol followed by injection of paclitaxel.[33] Mild pancreatitis and splenic vein obliteration were reported in the study.

These preliminary studies highlight the technical feasibility and safety of EUS-guided ethanol ablation of pancreatic cystic tumors which can be considered in patients who are not good surgical candidates or who refuse surgery, in an asymptomatic cystic lesion that has increased in size on follow-up study and in case of benign appearing and morphologically indeterminate cysts.[34] However, randomized controlled prospective trials are needed to evaluate the clinical efficacy and safety of this technique. Until further data are available, this therapy should be used with caution in carefully selected patient populations.

EUS-guided ethanol ablation of pancreatic neuroendocrine tumor has also been reported.[35] EUS-guided ethanol ablation of a 13-mm insulinoma has been reported in a 78-year-old woman who was a poor surgical candidate. A single injection of 8 mL 95% ethanol was injected into the tumor, resulting in complete remission of the tumor and of the recurrent symptomatic hypoglycemia. Levy and colleagues[36] in 2012 retrospectively reviewed 8 patients with insulinoma, managed with ultrasound-guided ethanol ablation. EUS-guided ethanol ablation was performed in 5 of those patients with complete resolution of hypoglycemia-related symptoms. No complications were reported during or after the EUS procedure. These cases reveal that EUS-guided ethanol ablation can be used for pancreatic neuroendocrine tumors for patients who refuse surgery or who are poor surgical candidates. EUS-guided ethanol ablation has also been reported in a 59-year-old man who was found to have a 4-cm gastric gastrointestinal stromal tumor (GIST) in the muscularis propria.[37] Because the patient was a poor surgical candidate, the lesion was treated with EUS-guided injection of 1.5 mL 95% ethanol. At 7 weeks' follow-up, no residual tumor was seen on EUS but a 1.5-cm ulcer was seen that resolved with treatment by acid suppression.

EUS-guided alcohol ablation of a 5-cm left adrenal gland metastasis from non-small cell lung cancer has been reported.[38] EUS-guided alcohol ablation of solid hepatic metastasis[39] and metastatic pelvic lymph nodes in a patient with rectal cancer[40] have been reported in the literature.

The technique of EUS-FNI with ethanol ablation continues to evolve; however, larger studies are needed to better understand the safety and efficacy of this technique.

EUS-guided Delivery of Antitumor Agents

A variety of agents have been used for EUS-guided local treatment of pancreatic cancer. Some of these agents (immature dendritic cells [DC], mixed lymphocyte culture [cytoimplant], and oncolytic virus) are discussed in this section.

- Immature DC–These are antigen-presenting cells that stimulate naive T lymphocytes into tumor-specific cytolytic cells. Akiyama and colleagues[41] presented the first results of DC-based therapy against syngeneic hamster pancreatic cancer and reported a growth inhibition rate of 82%. In 2007, Irisawa and colleagues[42] conducted an EUS-guided injection of immature DC in 7 patients with advanced pancreatic cancer with prior chemotherapy failure. Before the initial DC injection, 5 of the 7 patients underwent irradiation to maximize antigen exposure by causing tumor necrosis. Median patient survival was noted to be 9.9 months[42] in the study with no procedure-related complications. No clinical toxicity with the DC injection was reported. Additional studies are needed to evaluate efficacy of this technique.
- Cytoimplant (Allogenic Mixed Lymphocyte Culture)–Chang and colleagues[43] used cytoimplant and injected these conjugates into pancreatic cancer locally under EUS guidance. The study was conducted in 8 patients with unresectable pancreatic adenocarcinoma and doses were given in escalating fashion (3, 6, or 9 billion cells) by a single EUS-guided FNI. No major complications

were reported except transient gastrointestinal toxicity and transient hyperbilirubinemia in 3 patients that was managed by replacement of biliary stents. Eighty-six percent of patients developed a low-grade fever. Two of the 8 patients had a partial response in tumor size and one had a minor response. Median survival of 13.2 months was reported in the study. This phase I clinical trial reported feasibility without any substantial toxicity of single injection cytoimplant immunotherapy by EUS-FNI in patients with unresectable pancreatic cancer. Larger studies are needed to further evaluate the efficacy and safety of this modality.

- Oncolytic Virus Therapy ONYX-015: Oncolytic viruses such as adenovirus and herpes virus have been studied for antitumor therapy in pancreatic cancer using EUS-FNI. A replication-selective virus preferentially replicates in tumor cells and destroys them from the inside, thus leading to spread into the neighboring cells. ONYX-015 is the first of these viruses given by EUS-guided injection in clinical trials. Mulvihill and colleagues[44] in 2001 reported CT-guided ONYX-015 injection in patients with pancreatic cancer. A minor response was reported in 6 of 22 patients. A CT-guided approach is however difficult because of the requirement of multiple percutaneous injections. Hecht and colleagues[45] performed EUS-guided ONYX-015 injection, in combination with gemcitabine, in 21 patients with 8 injections over a period of 8 weeks. Two patients had partial regression of the injected tumor and two patients had a minor response. Six patients had stable disease and 11 had progressive disease or had to be dropped from the study due to treatment toxicity. Complication rates were higher compared with previous studies. Two patients had sepsis before the institution of prophylactic antibiotics in the study and 2 patients had duodenal perforations leading to subsequent change in the protocol of performing transgastric injections only. This study reports feasibility of EUS-guided ONYX-015 injection into pancreatic cancer using a transgastric route.
- TNFerade injection: TNFerade is a replication deficient adenovector, which contains a radiation-inducible promoter carrying the human tumor necrosis factor (TNF) -α gene. Chang and colleagues[46,47] have evaluated EUS-guided TNFerade in patients with locally advanced pancreatic cancer. In a phase I/II study Hecht and colleagues[48]

evaluated the efficacy of TNFerade combined with IV chemotherapy (5-Fluorouracil) and radiation. Patients with locally advanced pancreatic cancer received weekly EUS-guided or percutaneous-guided injection of TNFerade (4×10^9, 4×10^{10}, 4×10^{11}, and 1×10^{12} particle units in 2 mL) for 5 weeks in conjunction with chemotherapy and radiation. Fifty patients were enrolled in the study and results revealed that toxicity related to TNFerade was seen at higher doses, making 4×10^{11} particle units (PU) the maximum tolerated dose. Three patients in the 1×10^{12} particle units group had pancreatitis and cholangitis. Patients receiving 4×10^{11} PU had a longer median survival compared with the other groups. Thus, patients receiving higher doses were seen to have better locoregional disease control, median survival, and higher chance of resective surgery after combination treatment.[46–48]

Although EUS-guided antitumor agents seem promising, larger phase III randomized controlled trials are needed to evaluate the efficacy of this technique further.

EUS-guided Bile Duct Access

Endoscopic retrograde cholangiopancreatography (ERCP) is usually the procedure of choice for alleviating bile duct obstruction resulting from locally advanced pancreatic cancer or cholangiocarcinoma. In patients with difficult anatomy from prior interventions, Whipple procedure, prior hepaticojejunostomy, Billroth II anatomy, or due to locally advanced pancreatic, ampullary, or biliary tumors obstructing the duodenum, conventional ERCP may not be successful via the transpapillary approach. Alternatives include percutaneous transhepatic cholangiography, which may lead to complications like recurrent cholangitis, bleeding, and fistula formation. Thus in patients where transpapillary access to the bile duct fails, EUS-guided biliary access can be achieved from the left intrahepatic system (transgastric approach) or by accessing the extrahepatic common bile duct (CBD) from the duodenum (Fig. 3). In either case, the final access can be transpapillary or transluminal.

In the transpapillary approach, under EUS guidance, the bile duct is accessed using a 19-gauge or 22-gauge needle. Once confirmed with cholangiogram, a 0.035-inch guidewire is then passed through the FNA needle tract. Efforts are made to advance the guidewire across the stricture allowing passage of the wire from the ampulla fo transpapillary stent placement using the standa

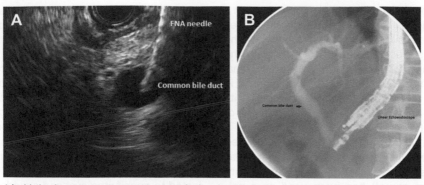

Fig. 3. EUS-guided bile duct access in a patient with distal CBD obstruction. (*A*) EUS-guided transduodenal puncture of common bile duct with FNA needle. (*B*) Contrast injected into CBD through the FNA needle.

ERCP approach. This EUS-guided "Rendezvous" technique is thought to be safer than placing a transluminal biliary stent through the stomach or duodenum. When the transpapillary stenting is unsuccessful, the transgastric or transduodenal access tract is dilated using a balloon dilator followed by placement of a plastic or self-expanding metal biliary stent.

EUS-guided choledochoduodenostomy, described in multiple case series, has a pooled technical success rate of 83% with a major complication rate of 10% to 15%, such as pneumoperitoneum, hemorrhage, cholangitis, pancreatitis, bile peritonitis, biloma, and duodenal perforation.[1] The transhepatic technique has been reported to have a pooled technical success of 73% with a 10% to 15% complication rate.[1] These procedures are technically challenging and should be reserved for carefully selected patients and performed at an expert center after detailed informed consent. Further studies are needed to better delineate the clinical efficacy, safety of these techniques, and standardization of these procedures.

EUS-guided Tumor Ablation

EUS-guided FNI has opened multiple avenues for local ablation of gastrointestinal tumors and cysts. Local ablation therapy has the potential to reduce tumor volume, thereby potentially impacting pain and local tumor-related complications and overall quality of life.

- Photodynamic therapy (PDT)–involves the principle of tumor localization by systemic administration of a photosensitizing agent and then tissue exposure by flexible fiber optics, which delivers light of appropriate wavelength. Photosensitizers (injected intravenously before the procedure) accumulate preferentially in the tumors than in normal tissue. The PDT fiber is introduced via a 19-gauge

EUS-FNA needle that leads to generation of highly reactive oxygen species called singlet oxygen, which in turn causes direct tumor cell destruction, induction of local inflammation, and damage to the tumor vasculature.[49] Bown and colleagues[50] have reported percutaneous CT-guided PDT of inoperable adenocarcinoma of the head of the pancreas in 16 patients. Localized necrosis was seen in all patients and none had clinical evidence of pancreatitis. Also, no treatment-related mortality was reported. EUS-guided PDT has been reported in a porcine model[51,52] and both studies found localized pancreatic necrosis without any significant complications.

- Radiofrequency ablation (RFA)–uses the principle of delivering thermal injury to the targeted tissue using electromagnetic energy, thus leading to cellular damage by inducing coagulation necrosis. It has been used in patients with hepatocellular cancer and metastatic hepatic carcinoma with a more than 90% success rate.[53] RFA of unresectable pancreatic head cancer has been reported using percutaneous, open, or laparoscopic approach. However, this has been associated with significant morbidity and 25% mortality from gastrointestinal bleeding and acute renal failure in one study.[54,55] In 1999 Goldberg and colleagues[56] first reported the application of EUS-guided RFA in a porcine model. EUS-guided ablation may pose lesser risk than conventional methods because it is less invasive and provides real-time imaging. Carrara and colleagues[57] used a hybrid bipolar probe combined with cryotechnology in a porcine model. They found the extent of the ablation area to be related to the duration of application with lesser complications than conventional techniques of RFA. A recent study by Gaidhane and colleagues[58] evaluated a prototype RFA probe adjusted to fit through a 19-gauge FNA needle in the porcine model. Greater tissue injury was found in the pancreas closer to the procedure site. The procedure was well tolerated with minimal pancreatitis. Further studies are required in humans to evaluate the safety and feasibility of EUS-guided RFA in the management of pancreatic cancer.

- Nd:YAG laser and high-intensity focused ultrasound (HIFU)–Percutaneous laser ablation using Nd:YAG (neodymium:yttrium aluminum garnet) has been used as a palliative therapy in hepatocellular carcinoma, malignant thyroid nodules, and hepatic metastasis.[59–61] In a study in a porcine model using EUS-guided Nd:YAG laser, tissue necrosis was seen in all 8 pigs with no major postprocedural complications.[62] A case of EUS-guided ablation of hepatocellular carcinoma in the caudate lobe using Nd:YAG laser has been reported.[63] HIFU is being widely used for noninvasive ablation of hepatic tumors.[64,65] Hwang and colleagues[66] developed a new HIFU transducer with the ability to attach to the EUS scope and thereby they could successfully create ablation in porcine liver and pancreas. Further large studies evaluating the safety and feasibility of these techniques are needed.

Pancreatic Pseudocyst and Pelvic Abscess Drainage with the Aid of EUS

EUS-guided pancreatic pseudocyst drainage

Pancreatic fluid collections could develop as a sequela of trauma, acute or chronic pancreatitis, or surgery. Complicated and symptomatic pancreatic pseudocysts can be drained surgically, radiologically, and endoscopically. With the help of EUS, in carefully selected patients, transmural drainage of the pseudocyst into the stomach or duodenum can be performed. EUS allows measuring the distance of the pseudocyst from the bowel wall, determining the presence of any intervening blood vessels, and also distinguishing a pseudocyst from walled-off necrosis. EUS also helps determine the optimal site for needle puncture in cysts which do not create an internal bulge into the gut wall.

In 2 prospective randomized trials, the transmural technique of EUS-guided pseudocyst drainage has been shown to be superior to the non-EUS approach.[67,68] Technical success of EUS-guided pseudocyst drainage has been reported to be greater than 90% in multiple studies.[67,69,70] Complications of this procedure include perforation, air

embolism, bleeding, stent migration, and systemic infections. Complication rates up to 30% have been reported.[70–72] In a study of 148 patients undergoing EUS-guided cyst drainage, Varadarajulu and colleagues[71] reported an infection rate of 2.7%, bleeding and stent migration rate of 0.67%, and perforation rate of 1.3%. A higher perforation rate was seen with drainage of an uncinate process fluid collection when compared with fluid collections in other pancreatic locations.[71] Under EUS guidance, the optimal puncture site is selected and the cyst is punctured. Contrast is injected to opacify the cyst and a guidewire is introduced into the cyst. The tract is dilated using a bougie, needle knife, or dilation balloon. A stent is then placed to allow for transgastric or transduodenal drainage of the cyst. Double pigtail plastic stents are usually used but the use of covered metal stents has also been reported in draining cysts of indeterminate adherence.[69,73]

Fig. 4 demonstrates the endoscopic drainage of pancreatic pseudocyst under EUS guidance. Nasocystic drains can also be placed in addition to endoprosthesis with a high success rate.[74] EUS-guided endoscopic necrosectomy has also been performed with an approximately 80% clinical success rate.[72,75] Thus, in carefully selected patients and in the hands of experienced endoscopists, these techniques can be used in an effective manner.

EUS-guided pelvic abscess drainage

Drainage of a pelvic abscess can be complex because of difficult anatomy. Rectal EUS has been successfully performed to provide internal drainage of pelvic abscesses not amenable to CT-guided drainage.[76] Successful drainage has also been reported with internal stent placement for abscess drainage with placement of a transrectal drainage catheter that is used for irrigation. This technique may enable a shorter hospital stay and minimize the risk of dislodgment of the drainage catheter.[77] A study of EUS-guided drainage and stenting of postoperative intra-abdominal and pelvic fluid collections in oncologic surgery reported internal drainage of perigastric abscess, perigastric hematoma, rectal hematoma, perirectal biloma, and perirectal abscess. The EUS approach allows access to difficult-to-reach anatomic areas, which are not easily accessible by CT-guided approach. Also, internal drainage of the abscess offers more patient comfort.[78] No major complications have been reported with EUS-guided abscess drainage in multiple studies.[79,80] Thus, EUS provides a safe, effective, and minimally invasive approach for internal drainage of abdominal-pelvic abscesses in carefully selected patients.

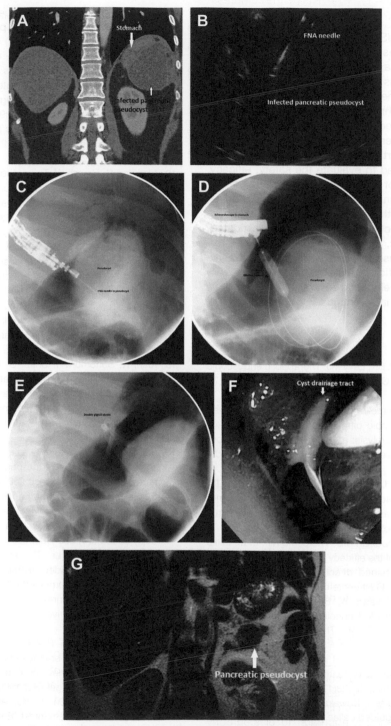

Fig. 4. Pancreatic pseudocyst drainage under EUS guidance. (*A*) CT revealing a large infected pancreatic pseudocyst compressing the stomach. (*B*) Transgastric puncture of the pancreatic pseudocyst with a 19-gauge needle. (*C*) Contrast injected into the pseudocyst and the cyst is opacified. (*D*) Balloon dilation of the cyst puncture tract. (*E*) Transgastric double pigtail stents placed into the cyst to facilitate drainage. (*F*) Pus draining from the cyst into the stomach. (*G*) MR imaging 2 weeks later revealing significant decrease in size of the pseudocyst.

SUMMARY

In summary, EUS technology has evolved over the last few decades from a diagnostic modality to one that serves as a platform for multiple therapeutic interventions, as detailed above.

A few of the above-mentioned EUS-guided therapeutic techniques (eg, antitumor agent injection, EUS-guided ablation, and EUS-guided brachytherapy) seem promising in selected patients with cancer. Further large prospective randomized trials are needed to evaluate the safety, efficacy, and feasibility of these interventions. Some newer techniques such as EUS-guided treatment of gastric varices with combined coiling and cyanoacrylate glue injection are also being investigated. In this dynamic, constantly evolving field of interventional endoscopy, newer minimally invasive therapeutic options for patients with cancer will continue to develop, and several of these will likely be EUS-based interventions.

REFERENCES

1. Abu Dayyeh BK, Levy MJ. Therapeutic endoscopic ultrasound. Gastroenterol Hepatol (N Y) 2012;8(7): 450–6.
2. Sahai AV, Lemelin V, Lam E, et al. Central vs bilateral endoscopic ultrasound-guided celiac plexus block or neurolysis: a comparative study of short-term effectiveness. Am J Gastroenterol 2009;104: 326–9.
3. Sakamoto H, Kitano M, Kamata K, et al. EUS-guided broad plexus neurolysis over the superior mesenteric artery using a 25-gauge needle. Am J Gastroenterol 2010;105(12):2599–606.
4. Levy MJ, Topazian MD, Wiersema MJ, et al. Initial evaluation of the efficacy and safety of endoscopic ultrasound-guided direct Ganglia neurolysis and block. Am J Gastroenterol 2008;103(1):98–103.
5. Suzuki R, Irisawa A, Bhutani MS. Endoscopic ultrasound-guided oncologic therapy for pancreatic cancer. Diagn Ther Endosc 2013;2013: 157581.
6. Wallace MB, Hawes RH. Endoscopic ultrasound in the evaluation and treatment of chronic pancreatitis. Pancreas 2001;23(1):26–35.
7. Doi S, Yasuda I, Kawakami H, et al. Endoscopic ultrasound-guided celiac ganglia neurolysis vs. celiac plexus neurolysis: a randomized multicenter trial. Endoscopy 2013;45(5):362–9.
8. Kaufman M, Singh G, Das S, et al. Efficacy of endoscopic ultrasound-guided celiac plexus block and celiac plexus neurolysis for managing abdominal pain associated with chronic pancreatitis and pancreatic cancer. J Clin Gastroenterol 2010; 44(2):127–34.
9. Yan BM, Myers RP. Neurolytic celiac plexus block for pain control in unresectable pancreatic cancer. Am J Gastroenterol 2007;102(2):430–8.
10. Gress F, Schmitt C, Sherman S, et al. Endoscopic ultrasound-guided celiac plexus block for managing abdominal pain associated with chronic pancreatitis: a prospective single center experience. Am J Gastroenterol 2001;96(2):409–16.
11. Hoffman BJ. EUS-guided celiac plexus block/neurolysis. Gastrointest Endosc 2002;56(Suppl 4): S26–8.
12. Mahajan R, Nowell W, Theerathorn P, et al. Empyema after endoscopic ultrasound guided celiac plexus pain block in chronic pancreatitis. Experience at an academic center. Gastrointest Endosc 2002;55:AB101.
13. Gimeno-Garcia AZ, Elwassief A, Paquin SC, et al. Fatal complication after endoscopic ultrasound-guided celiac plexus neurolysis. Endoscopy 2012;44(Suppl 2 UCTN):E267.
14. Zhongmin W, Yu L, Fenju L, et al. Clinical efficacy of CT-guided iodine-125 seed implantation therapy in patients with advanced pancreatic cancer. Eur Radiol 2010;20(7):1786–91.
15. Kishi K, Sonomura T, Shirai S, et al. Brachytherapy reirradiation with hyaluronate gel injection of paraaortic lymphnode metastasis of pancreatic cancer: paravertebral approach–a technical report with a case. J Radiat Res 2011;52(6): 840–4.
16. Sun S, Qingjie L, Qiyong G, et al. EUS-guided interstitial brachytherapy of the pancreas: a feasibility study. Gastrointest Endosc 2005;62(5):775–9.
17. Sun S, Xu H, Xin J, et al. Endoscopic ultrasound-guided interstitial brachytherapy of unresectable pancreatic cancer: results of a pilot trial. Endoscopy 2006;38(4):399–403.
18. Jin Z, Du Y, Li Z, et al. Endoscopic ultrasonography-guided interstitial implantation of iodine 125-seeds combined with chemotherapy in the treatment of unresectable pancreatic carcinoma: a prospective pilot study. Endoscopy 2008;40(4):314–20.
19. Maier W, Henne K, Krebs A, et al. Endoscopic ultrasound-guided brachytherapy of head and neck tumours. A new procedure for controlled application. J Laryngol Otol 1999;113(1):41–8.
20. Lah JJ, Kuo JV, Chang KJ, et al. EUS-guided brachytherapy. Gastrointest Endosc 2005;62(5): 805–8.
21. Pishvaian AC, Collins B, Gagnon G, et al. EUS-guided fiducial placement for CyberKnife radiotherapy of mediastinal and abdominal malignancies. Gastrointest Endosc 2006;64(3):412–7.
22. Al-Haddad M, Eloubeidi MA. Interventional EUS for the diagnosis and treatment of locally advanced pancreatic cancer. JOP 2010;11(1):1–7.

23. Majumder S, Berzin TM, Mahadevan A, et al. Endoscopic ultrasound-guided pancreatic fiducial placement: how important is ideal fiducial geometry? Pancreas 2013;42(4):692–5.

24. Olender D. Fiducials for target localization. In: Heilbrun MP, editor. Cyberknife radiosurgery: a practical guide. Sunnyvale (CA): Cyberknife Society; 2003. p. 80–94.

25. Omerovic S, Zerem E. Alcohol sclerotherapy in the treatment of symptomatic simple renal cysts. Bosn J Basic Med Sci 2008;8(4):337–40.

26. Larssen TB, Jensen DK, Viste A, et al. Single-session alcohol sclerotherapy in symptomatic benign hepatic cysts. Long-term results. Acta Radiol 1999;40(6):636–8.

27. Livraghi T, Bolondi L, Lazzaroni S, et al. Percutaneous ethanol injection in the treatment of hepatocellular carcinoma in cirrhosis. A study on 207 patients. Cancer 1992;69(4):925–9.

28. Xiao YY, Tian JL, Li JK, et al. CT-guided percutaneous chemical ablation of adrenal neoplasms. AJR Am J Roentgenol 2008;190(1):105–10.

29. Aslanian H, Salem RR, Marginean C, et al. EUS-guided ethanol injection of normal porcine pancreas: a pilot study. Gastrointest Endosc 2005;62(5):723–7.

30. Gan SI, Thompson CC, Lauwers GY, et al. Ethanol lavage of pancreatic cystic lesions: initial pilot study. Gastrointest Endosc 2005; 61(6):746–52.

31. DeWitt J, McGreevy K, Schmidt CM, et al. EUS-guided ethanol versus saline solution lavage for pancreatic cysts: a randomized, double-blind study. Gastrointest Endosc 2009; 70(4):710–23.

32. Oh HC, Seo DW, Lee TY, et al. New treatment for cystic tumors of the pancreas: EUS-guided ethanol lavage with paclitaxel injection. Gastrointest Endosc 2008;67(4):636–42.

33. Oh HC, Seo DW, Song TJ, et al. Endoscopic ultrasonography-guided ethanol lavage with paclitaxel injection treats patients with pancreatic cysts. Gastroenterology 2011;140(1):172–9.

34. Zhang WY, Li ZS, Jin ZD. Endoscopic ultrasound-guided ethanol ablation therapy for tumors. World J Gastroenterol 2013;19(22):3397–403.

35. Jurgensen C, Schuppan D, Neser F, et al. EUS-guided alcohol ablation of an insulinoma. Gastrointest Endosc 2006;63(7):1059–62.

36. Levy MJ, Thompson GB, Topazian MD, et al. US-guided ethanol ablation of insulinomas: a new treatment option. Gastrointest Endosc 2012;75(1):200–6.

37. Gunter E, Lingenfelser T, Eitelbach F, et al. EUS-guided ethanol injection for treatment of a GI stromal tumor. Gastrointest Endosc 2003;57(1):113–5.

38. Artifon EL, Lucon AM, Sakai P, et al. EUS-guided alcohol ablation of left adrenal metastasis from non-small-cell lung carcinoma. Gastrointest Endosc 2007;66(6):1201–5.

39. Barclay RL, Perez-Miranda M, Giovannini M. EUS-guided treatment of a solid hepatic metastasis. Gastrointest Endosc 2002;55(2):266–70.

40. DeWitt J, Mohamadnejad M. EUS-guided alcohol ablation of metastatic pelvic lymph nodes after endoscopic resection of polypoid rectal cancer: the need for long-term surveillance. Gastrointest Endosc 2011;74(2):446–7.

41. Akiyama Y, Maruyama K, Nara N, et al. Antitumor effects induced by dendritic cell-based immunotherapy against established pancreatic cancer in hamsters. Cancer Lett 2002;184(1):37–47.

42. Irisawa A, Takagi T, Kanazawa M, et al. Endoscopic ultrasound-guided fine-needle injection of immature dendritic cells into advanced pancreatic cancer refractory to gemcitabine: a pilot study. Pancreas 2007;35(2):189–90.

43. Chang KJ, Nguyen PT, Thompson JA, et al. Phase I clinical trial of allogeneic mixed lymphocyte culture (cytoimplant) delivered by endoscopic ultrasound-guided fine-needle injection in patients with advanced pancreatic carcinoma. Cancer 2000; 88(6):1325–35.

44. Mulvihill S, Warren R, Venook A, et al. Safety and feasibility of injection with an E1B-55 kDa gene-deleted, replication-selective adenovirus (ONYX-015) into primary carcinomas of the pancreas: a phase I trial. Gene Ther 2001;8(4):308–15.

45. Hecht JR, Bedford R, Abbruzzese JL, et al. A phase I/II trial of intratumoral endoscopic ultrasound injection of ONYX-015 with intravenous gemcitabine in unresectable pancreatic carcinoma. Clin Cancer Res 2003;9(2):555–61.

46. Chang KJ, Irisawa A, Group EUSW. EUS 2008 Working Group document: evaluation of EUS-guided injection therapy for tumors. Gastrointest Endosc 2009;69(Suppl 2):S54–8.

47. Chang KJ, Lee JG, Holcombe RF, et al. Endoscopic ultrasound delivery of an antitumor agent to treat a case of pancreatic cancer. Nat Clin Pract Gastroenterol Hepatol 2008;5(2):107–11.

48. Hecht JR, Farrell JJ, Senzer N, et al. EUS or percutaneously guided intratumoral TNFerade biologic with 5-fluorouracil and radiotherapy for first-line treatment of locally advanced pancreatic cancer: a phase I/II study. Gastrointest Endosc 2012; 75(2):332–8.

49. Agostinis P, Berg K, Cengel KA, et al. Photodynamic therapy of cancer: an update. CA Cancer J Clin 2011;61(4):250–81.

50. Bown SG, Rogowska AZ, Whitelaw DE, et al. Photodynamic therapy for cancer of the pancreas. Gut 2002;50(4):549–57.

51. Chan HH, Nishioka NS, Mino M, et al. EUS-guided photodynamic therapy of the pancreas: a pilot study. Gastrointest Endosc 2004;59(1):95–9.

52. Yusuf TE, Matthes K, Brugge WR. EUS-guided photodynamic therapy with verteporfin for ablation of normal pancreatic tissue: a pilot study in a porcine model (with video). Gastrointest Endosc 2008;67(6):957–61.

53. Chen MH, Yang W, Yan K, et al. Treatment efficacy of radiofrequency ablation of 338 patients with hepatic malignant tumor and the relevant complications. World J Gastroenterol 2005; 11(40):6395–401.

54. Wu Y, Tang Z, Fang H, et al. High operative risk of cool-tip radiofrequency ablation for unresectable pancreatic head cancer. J Surg Oncol 2006; 94(5):392–5.

55. Spiliotis JD, Datsis AC, Michalopoulos NV, et al. High operative risk of cool-tip radiofrequency ablation for unresectable pancreatic head cancer. J Surg Oncol 2007;96(1):89–90.

56. Goldberg SN, Mallery S, Gazelle GS, et al. EUS-guided radiofrequency ablation in the pancreas: results in a porcine model. Gastrointest Endosc 1999;50(3):392–401.

57. Carrara S, Arcidiacono PG, Albarello L, et al. Endoscopic ultrasound-guided application of a new hybrid cryotherm probe in porcine pancreas: a preliminary study. Endoscopy 2008;40(4):321–6.

58. Gaidhane M, Smith I, Ellen K, et al. Endoscopic ultrasound-guided radiofrequency ablation (EUS-RFA) of the pancreas in a porcine model. Gastroenterol Res Pract 2012;2012:431451.

59. Pacella CM, Francica G, Di Lascio FM, et al. Long-term outcome of cirrhotic patients with early hepatocellular carcinoma treated with ultrasound-guided percutaneous laser ablation: a retrospective analysis. J Clin Oncol 2009;27(16):2615–21.

60. Pacella CM, Bizzarri G, Spiezia S, et al. Thyroid tissue: US-guided percutaneous laser thermal ablation. Radiology 2004;232(1):272–80.

61. Vogl TJ, Straub R, Eichler K, et al. Colorectal carcinoma metastases in liver: laser-induced interstitial thermotherapy–local tumor control rate and survival data. Radiology 2004;230(2):450–8.

62. Di Matteo F, Martino M, Rea R, et al. EUS-guided Nd:YAG laser ablation of normal pancreatic tissue: a pilot study in a pig model. Gastrointest Endosc 2010;72(2):358–63.

63. Di Matteo F, Grasso R, Pacella CM, et al. EUS-guided Nd:YAG laser ablation of a hepatocellular carcinoma in the caudate lobe. Gastrointest Endosc 2011;73(3):632–6.

64. Kim J, Chung DJ, Jung SE, et al. Therapeutic effect of high-intensity focused ultrasound combined with transarterial chemoembolisation for hepatocellular carcinoma <5 cm: comparison with transarterial chemoembolisation monotherapy–preliminary observations. Br J Radiol 2012; 85(1018):e940–6.

65. Leslie T, Ritchie R, Illing R, et al. High-intensity focused ultrasound treatment of liver tumours: post-treatment MRI correlates well with intra-operative estimates of treatment volume. Br J Radiol 2012;85(1018):1363–70.

66. Hwang J, Farr N, Morrison K, et al. Development of an EUS-guided high-intensity focused ultrasound endoscope. Gastrointest Endosc 2011;73(4S): AB155.

67. Varadarajulu S, Christein JD, Tamhane A, et al. Prospective randomized trial comparing EUS and EGD for transmural drainage of pancreatic pseudocysts (with videos). Gastrointest Endosc 2008; 68(6):1102–11.

68. Park DH, Lee SS, Moon SH, et al. Endoscopic ultrasound-guided versus conventional transmural drainage for pancreatic pseudocysts: a prospective randomized trial. Endoscopy 2009;41(10): 842–8.

69. Varadarajulu S, Tamhane A, Blakely J. Graded dilation technique for EUS-guided drainage of peripancreatic fluid collections: an assessment of outcomes and complications and technical proficiency (with video). Gastrointest Endosc 2008; 68(4):656–66.

70. Lopes CV, Pesenti C, Bories E, et al. Endoscopic-ultrasound-guided endoscopic transmural drainage of pancreatic pseudocysts and abscesses. Scand J Gastroenterol 2007;42(4):524–9.

71. Varadarajulu S, Christein JD, Wilcox CM. Frequency of complications during EUS-guided drainage of pancreatic fluid collections in 148 consecutive patients. J Gastroenterol Hepatol 2011;26(10):1504–8.

72. Seewald S, Ang TL, Richter H, et al. Long-term results after endoscopic drainage and necrosectomy of symptomatic pancreatic fluid collections. Dig Endosc 2012;24:36–41.

73. Weilert F, Binmoeller KF, Shah JN, et al. Endoscopic ultrasound-guided drainage of pancreatic fluid collections with indeterminate adherence using temporary covered metal stents. Endoscopy 2012;44(8):780–3.

74. Puri R, Mishra SR, Thandassery RB, et al. Outcome and complications of endoscopic ultrasound guided pancreatic pseudocyst drainage using combined endoprosthesis and naso-cystic drain. J Gastroenterol Hepatol 2012;27(4):722–7.

75. Seifert H, Biermer M, Schmitt W, et al. Transluminal endoscopic necrosectomy after acute pancreatitis: a multicentre study with long-term follow-up (the GEPARD Study). Gut 2009;58(9):1260–6.

76. Puri R, Eloubeidi MA, Sud R, et al. Endoscopic ultrasound-guided drainage of pelvic abscess

without fluoroscopy guidance. J Gastroenterol Hepatol 2010;25(8):1416–9.

77. Trevino JM, Drelichman ER, Varadarajulu S. Modified technique for EUS-guided drainage of pelvic abscess (with video). Gastrointest Endosc 2008; 68(6):1215–9.

78. Ulla-Rocha JL, Vilar-Cao Z, Sardina-Ferreiro R. EUS-guided drainage and stent placement for postoperative intra-abdominal and pelvic fluid collections in oncological surgery. Therap Adv Gastroenterol 2012;5(2):95–102.

79. Giovannini M, Bories E, Moutardier V, et al. Drainage of deep pelvic abscesses using therapeutic echo endoscopy. Endoscopy 2003;35(6):511–4.

80. Varadarajulu S, Drelichman ER. Effectiveness of EUS in drainage of pelvic abscesses in 25 consecutive patients (with video). Gastrointest Endosc 2009;70(6):1121–7.

Ultrasound Guidance in Tumor Ablation

Joseph Reis, MD*, Devang Butani, MD

KEYWORDS

- Ultrasound guidance • Ablation • Tumor • Radiofrequency • Cryoablation • Liver • Kidney

KEY POINTS

- Ultrasonography is increasingly being used during the targeting phase of ablation procedures.
- Contrast-enhanced ultrasonography and sonoelastography have significantly improved lesion visualization before, during, and after ablation.
- The use of various imaging modalities and ablative techniques is encouraged to allow appropriate individualization of treatment.
- Ultrasonography will be used in the future to aid irreversible electroporation and microwave ablation as these techniques gain in popularity.

INTRODUCTION

Ablation is a minimally invasive procedure used to treat both cancerous and noncancerous conditions. The International Group on Image-Guided Tumor ablation stressed, in their 2005 consensus statement, the "direct" nature of this therapy aimed at "eradication or substantial tumor destruction."[1] Applications for percutaneous ablation have broadly expanded since the initial treatment of hepatocellular carcinoma with percutaneous ethanol injection in 1986[2] largely due to improvements in technology, increased procedure availability, and mounting evidence that percutaneous ablation is equally effective to other oncologic treatments in the hands of an experienced operator. Alternative, and often coexisting, treatment options include chemoterapy, radiation, surgery, and transcatheter delivery of chemotherapy.

Methods of ablation vary in both their applications and mode of treatment. For example, radiofrequency ablation (RFA) may be applied to many different organ systems ranging from lung metastases to the osteoid osteomas. Most ablations performed by radiologists target the liver, kidneys, and lung. Understanding technical differences between modalities and target organs is essential to optimal treatment.

Ablative modalities are characterized as thermal, chemical, or electrical (Table 1). Each has advantages and disadvantages with respect to lesion size, location, and treatment intent. Thermal ablation induces cell death through the transmission of energy to water molecules, as in RFA, cryoablation, and microwave ablation. Chemical ablation refers to cell coagulation from the direct injection of a toxic agent such as alcohol. Electrical ablation techniques disrupt the cell-membrane electric gradient and thereby the inducing cell. The authors do not advocate strict adherence to one particular modality. The use of various modalities is encouraged to ensure optimal, individualized treatment options.

A comprehensive discussion of all ablative modalities is beyond the scope of this article. This review focuses on sonographic applications for 2 common methods of ablation, namely RFA and

The authors have nothing to disclose.
Division of Interventional Radiology, Department of Imaging Sciences, University of Rochester Medical Center, 601 Elmwood Avenue, Box 648, Rochester, NY 14642, USA
* Corresponding author.
E-mail address: Joseph_Reis@urmc.rochester.edu

Table 1
Types of ablation

Category	Ablative Technique
Chemical	Alcohol, acetic acid
Thermal	RFA, cryoablation, microwave, laser, HIFU
Electrical	IRE

Abbreviations: HIFU, high-intensity focused ultrasonography; IRE, irreversible electroporation; RFA, radiofrequency ablation.

cryoablation, in treating hepatic and renal tumors. Brief mention is given to microwave ablation and irreversible electroporation (IRE).

PRINCIPLES OF RADIOFREQUENCY ABLATION

RFA is based on the principle of vibrational energy transmission. Electromagnetic waves are transmitted to a probe that align water-molecule dipole moments. Alternating current is applied with subsequent shifts in alignment of the water molecules to the direction of current at a given time (**Fig. 1**). The rapid vibration of the molecules transmits thermal energy into cells.[3] Cell death is achieved when temperatures exceed 60°C. The optimal temperature range used during a procedure ranges from 60°C to 105°C. Above 105°C, cellular vaporization and charring occur that rapidly increase electrical resistance, decrease ablation

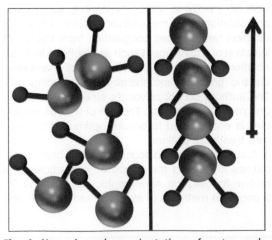

Fig. 1. Normal random orientation of water molecules within cells (*left*) and subsequent alignment of the negatively polarized oxygen molecules along the dipole moment (*right*). Molecules change direction with the shifting dipole moment of alternating current, producing vibrational energy. Red spheres indicate hydrogen, blue spheres oxygen.

times, shrink ablation zones, and thereby undertreat tumors.

Power requirements are dependent on the efficiency of energy transmission in vivo and the organ being targeted. Typical power ranges for generators applied to hepatic tumors are 150 to 250 W, whereas power requirements in the kidney are closer to 50 W.[4] The kidney is a smaller organ and lacks the dual blood supply present in the liver.

Probes used during the procedure deposit energy at their tips through a closed-loop circuit created using anode grounding pads attached to the patient. The probe may have a single tip or use metal tines that fan out from the probe tip. These tines are curvilinear and equidistant, forming an umbrella shape as they leave the probe, and determine the zone of ablation (**Fig. 2**). Complete deployment of the tines is necessary to ensure an adequate ablation zone diameter (see **Fig. 2**). Multiple probes with typical separation distances of approximately 1 cm may be used, which are internally cooled by instillation of a coolant during the procedure. Perfusion probes that allow injection of a solution into the tumor during the ablation are also available. **Box 1** summarizes the principles of RFA.

PRINCIPLES OF CRYOABLATION

Cryoablation is the induction of cell death by thermal conduction. Cell-membrane permeability and osmolar concentrations are drastically altered as intracellular and extracellular water molecules crystalize below −25°C. This process induces necrosis and apoptosis, and can cause surrounding dehydration and ischemia, particularly at temperatures lower than −40°C.[5]

Subzero cryoprobe temperatures are reached using the Joule-Thompson effect. Inert gases pass through a tiny opening in the probe to a large-volume chamber. The sudden increase in volume lowers the pressure and temperature of the gas, cooling the probe. Circulating coolant is used to complement heat exchange between the probe and surrounding tissue.[5] Up to 8 cryoprobes have been reported for use in a single session, geometrically oriented within 1 cm of the tumor and 2 cm of the nearest probe.[6] Probes used in cryoablation do not have tines. **Box 2** summarizes the principles of cryoablation.

GENERAL SELECTION CRITERIA

Patient selection, treatment intent, and tumor location are important considerations prior to the procedure. A multidisciplinary team

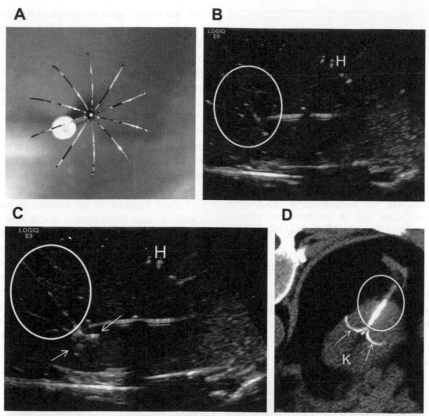

Fig. 2. Tines fan out from RFA probes like an umbrella (*A*), and deployment can be monitored continuously under US (*B, C*) or intermittently on cross-sectional imaging (*D*). Circle indicates probe and the arrows indicate tines. H, liver; K, kidney.

consisting of hepatologists, radiation oncologists, surgeons, diagnostic radiologists, and interventional radiologists are involved in treatment decisions, including the role of ablation. This comprehensive approach to patient care provides a forum for increased communication and education among physicians that leads to better outcomes. Once the patient has been selected for ablative treatment, a formal consultation is performed in the interventional radiology clinic. Images are reviewed with the patient, options are discussed, and potential complications are outlined. Poor performance status and quality of life are important considerations in decision

making, as they are significant prognostic factors in patient survival.[7]

Cross-sectional imaging is used to determine lesion accessibility and potential technical problems. The patient's complete blood count, international normalized ratio, prothrombin time (**Table 2**), and laboratory tests relevant to individual organ function, such as a liver functional panel, creatinine, and glomerular filtration rate, are obtained. Contraindications specific to RFA include the presence of an electrical stimulating device such as a pacemaker.

Additional selection criteria are specific to each organ.

Box 1
Principles of RFA

- Target temperature: 60°C to 105°C
- Heating method: alternating current
- Probes: maximum 5 probes; unipolar and bipolar; may contain tines

---

Box 2
Principles of cryoablation

- Target temperature: −25°C to −40°C
- Cooling method: Joule-Thompson effect
- Probes: maximum 8 probes; no tines

Table 2
Ablation periprocedural hematologic and coagulation parameters

Parameter	Accepted Standard
INR	<1.5
PTT	<1.5 × control
Platelets	>50,000/μL
Hematocrit	No consensus

Abbreviations: INR, international normalized ratio; PTT, partial thromboplastin time.
Data from Patel IJ, Davidson JC, Nikolic B, et al. Consensus guidelines for periprocedural coagulation status and hemostasis risk in percutaneous image-guided interventions. J Vasc Interv Radiol 2012;23:727–36.

SELECTION CRITERIA FOR HEPATIC ABLATION

Ablation of hepatocellular carcinoma is commonly reserved for primary treatment of small tumors 3 cm or less in diameter with a Barcelona Clinical Liver Stage 0 or A, treatment in individuals who are not candidates for surgical therapy based on performance status, palliation, and downstaging of isolated tumors larger than 5 cm or multiple tumors larger than 3 cm to bridge patients to transplantation.[8] Although small tumors can be treated surgically, as few as 15% of affected individuals are surgical candidates at the time of treatment.[9] Even patients with successful ablative treatment remain listed for transplantation due to the high rate of new tumor foci arising in a cirrhotic liver. Ablation can also be used to treat metastatic tumors that are limited in number and are 4 cm or less in diameter.[10]

Tumor location is an additional consideration. Lesions near intrahepatic ducts, the gallbladder, and extrahepatic organs such as the bowel or adrenal glands are difficult to treat considering the potential for damage to these structures during the procedure. In addition, nearby blood vessels can transfer thermal energy away from the tumor, known as the heat-sink effect (**Fig. 3**). This phenomenon can result in suboptimal heating of the tumor and inadequate treatment. Heat-sink effects

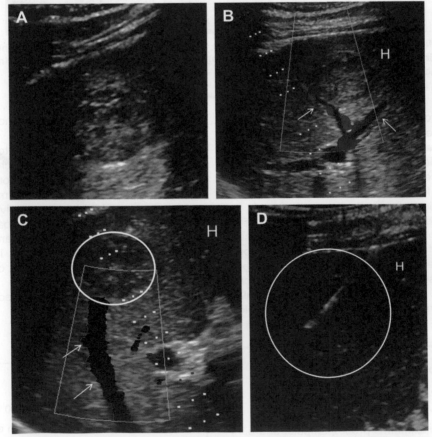

Fig. 3. Hepatic tumor detected on US (*A*), with good visualization of the adjacent hepatic arteries (*B*) and veins (*C*) before probe insertion (*D*). Arrows indicate hepatic arteries and veins, circle indicates mass and probe. H, liver.

also play a significant role in the kidney, which is highly vascular and diverts heat to the collecting system. **Box 3** summarizes the indications for hepatic ablation.

SELECTION CRITERIA FOR RENAL ABLATION

Ablation is directed at small renal masses of less than 4 cm that demonstrate growth over time or have suspicious imaging features. This procedure is nephron sparing, with efficacy rates comparable to those of partial nephrectomy, but shorter recovery and hospitalization times. Nephron-sparing surgery is particularly valuable in patients at high risk for recurrent malignancy, such as individuals suffering from Von Hippel–Lindau syndrome, patients with single kidneys, and those with renal insufficiency.

Both RFA and cryoablation are currently used to treat renal cell carcinoma. Both methods have comparable 5-year survival rates with upper limits of 87% to 97%.[11]

The optimal tumor is less than 4 cm in size, solid, and exophytic (**Fig. 4**). Therefore, treated tumors are typically TNM stage Ia. Complete ablation of tumors declines from greater than 90% to 25% as the tumor size increases to more than 5 cm.[12] Optimal ablation margins of 0.5 to 1 cm are more difficult to achieve with increasing size, and require the use of multiple probes. RFA is commonly performed with 1 or 2 probes that range in treatment diameter up to 5 cm, whereas cryoablation can be performed with multiple probes and diameters of ablation up to 4.0 × 6.7 cm depending on the manufacturer.[9] Cryoablation is typically chosen for lesions near the renal hilum because of its slightly lower complication rate.[13] Damage to the collecting system can also be prevented by instillation of a coolant solution into the pelvis through a renal stent.

Tumor composition is an additional complicating factor in ablation. Solid tumors have the best therapeutic response, whereas cystic tumors often require multiple separate ablation sessions for successful treatment. This difference has caused some to advocate for treatment of only

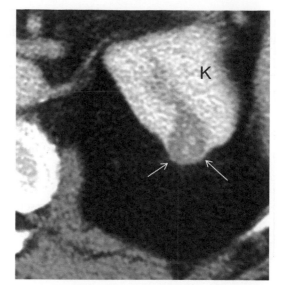

Fig. 4. The ideal location for a renal tumor is exophytic and posterior, surrounded by fat, away from other structures. Arrows indicate renal tumor. K, kidney.

those renal lesions with a solid component of 50% or greater.[12]

Exophytic location of tumors is desired to avoid damage to adjacent vital structures, such as the collecting system and blood vessels. RFA has lower efficacy near vessels because of the heat-sink effect discussed earlier. Indications for renal ablation are summarized in **Box 4**.

SELECTION OF IMAGING MODALITIES

Percutaneous ablation requires image guidance. Three imaging modalities are currently used to monitor intraprocedural ablation: computed tomography (CT), magnetic resonance imaging (MRI), and ultrasonography (US). Each modality has its advantages and disadvantages (**Table 3**). CT provides a large field of view and good visualization of cryoablation margins at the cost of ionizing radiation. MRI provides superior contrast resolution and detailed information about tissue temperatures (MR thermography) at the cost of extending imaging time and expensive compatible

---

Box 3
Indications for hepatic ablation

- Palliation
- Primary treatment (Barcelona 0 or A tumors)
- Bridge to transplantation
- Isolated metastases 4 cm or smaller

Box 4
Indications for renal ablation

- TNM Stage Ia tumor
- Nonoperative candidate
- Nephron-sparing surgery
- Refractory bleeding

Table 3
Advantages and disadvantages of imaging modalities

Modality	Advantages	Disadvantages
US	Real-time imaging Availability Low cost Lack of ionizing radiation	Limited field of view Limited depth Limited contrast resolution Shadowing artifacts
CT	Large field of view Good postcontrast resolution	Ionizing radiation No real-time imaging Limited noncontrast resolution Iodinated contrast agents Limited availability
MRI	Superior contrast resolution Adequate field of view Thermal tissue analysis	Extended procedure time Expensive compatible equipment Limited availability Motion sensitivity

ablation equipment. US provides the unique advantages of low cost, a lack of ionizing radiation, and real-time monitoring, but lacks a large field of view and adequate resolution at increasing lesion depth. Each modality also provides distinct advantages during individual stages of the ablation: planning, targeting, monitoring, controlling, and assessing treatment response.

CT and MRI are generally superior to US for the planning stages of the ablation. These modalities have a larger field of view, allowing for the detection of metastatic disease and direct tumor spread that could alter patient management. B-mode US can easily miss lesions that are isoechoic in patients with altered organ anatomy. Small tumor size, macronodular cirrhosis, subphrenic location of the lesion, obscuration from overlying structures such as ribs, and inaccurate probe-tip positioning are additional factors that limit visualization.[14,15] On rare occasions US may be able to detect lesions missed on CT, but this is not common.[16] US is particularly valuable in monitoring moving target lesions, such as tumors located in segments VII and VIII of the liver near the diaphragm. US can also detect solid components of complex cysts in patients who cannot have contrast, confirming their malignant histology (**Fig. 5**).

US is often used during probe insertion to target a lesion, given its real-time imaging (see **Fig. 3**). Although lesions can be missed on US, simultaneous CT imaging as well as sonoelastography and contrast-enhanced US (CEUS) serve as adjuncts to tumor detection. CT/MRI/US fusion has also been described in planning and targeting lesions for ablation, allowing for detection of 45% of previously undetectable tumors on US by using

a combination of fusion images and anatomic landmarks.[17]

CT and MRI are often superior to US during the monitoring phase of the procedure, owing to acoustic artifacts arising from the ablated tissue (**Fig. 6**). Initial sonographic images depict a hypoechoic area surrounding the zone of ablation. However, this area then becomes increasingly hyperechoic in RFA owing to the formation of small gas microbubbles within the treated tissue. These bubbles produce heterogeneity in the image that makes differentiation of treated tissue from normal tissue difficult. The presence of additional free gas formed during coagulation can result in "dirty" acoustic shadowing that obscures the leading edge of the tumor during treatment (see **Fig. 6**).[18] The development of long-acting contrast agents has since improved intraprocedural conspicuity of lesions.

US is similarly limited in detecting the leading edge of treatment during cryoablation (see **Fig. 6**). The ice ball formed in the procedure generates significant acoustic shadowing. Alternatively, CT produces a clear image of the ice ball with margins representing a temperature of 0°C (**Fig. 7**). Cell death occurs 3 mm deep to this boundary, allowing for comparison of preprocedure and postprocedure volumes to evaluate for adequate tumor treatment.

Postprocedure monitoring and follow-up may occur with any of the 3 modalities. Tumor recurrence is most commonly recognized as contrast enhancement from neovascularization. Contrast enhancement by US is equivalent to that of CT and MRI in the immediate postprocedural period, with the advantage of enhancing only the intravascular space.[19,20] However, US does not

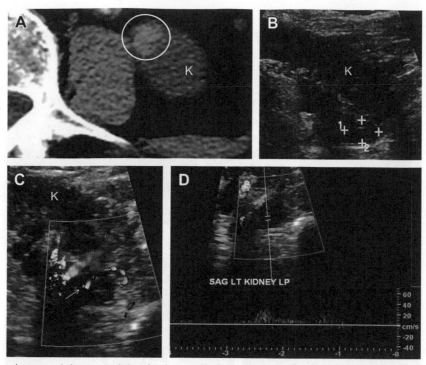

Fig. 5. A hyperdense nodule on CT (*A*) is further analyzed with gray-scale US (*B*), Doppler US (*C*), and spectral tracing (*D*) to demonstrate internal solid components. Circle/calipers indicate renal nodule; arrow indicates internal flow. K, kidney.

provide the same field of view for the detection of metastases.

SONOELASTOGRAPHY AND CONTRAST-ENHANCED ULTRASONOGRAPHY

Sonoelastography is a measurement of tissue displacement caused by perpendicular pressure forces. The sonographer applies cyclic compression over an area at a constant rate, generating a vibrational shear wave. Tissue displacement by a particular shear force is proportional to elastic modulus, and can help differentiate normal tissue from tumors (**Fig. 8**).[21] An alternative method is quasistatic compression, which produces strain forces on the tissue.[22] Tumors have high moduli that often vary between cell types and among individual cell histologies.

This method provides an accurate measurement of ablated tissue volume in 3-dimensional in vitro reconstructions of ablated tissue.[23] Ablated tissue is stiffer, allowing for good contrast resolution between ablated zones and normal parenchyma. However, limitations are present, including nonconsistent compression caused by probe slippage and differences in breathing. Additional ablation probes can be used in certain cases to provide a source for consistent compression.[24]

Contrast-enhanced US is sonographic imaging that follows the intravenous injection of microbubbles containing gas (**Fig. 9**). These microbubbles have diameters on the order of 40 μm and reflect ultrasound waves producing contrast resolution. Modern pulse-inversion imaging allows for contrast agents to be monitored over time without the problem of microbubble rupture initially experienced with CEUS.[25,26]

SPECIFICS OF ULTRASOUND-GUIDED PROCEDURES

Patients are brought into the imaging suite and positioned to optimize percutaneous access over the region of interest and to displace overlying structures. Shifting patient position from a supine to decubitus orientation may shift vital structures, such as the bowel, obstructing the target path. Patients treated for renal masses are often placed in the prone or decubitus position.

Initial imaging is then performed. US imaging may include a combination of B-mode, sonoelastography, and CEUS, depending on lesion conspicuity. Once the lesion is visualized and the overlying skin is sterilely cleaned and draped, sedation can be used. Fentanyl and midazolam provide adequate anesthesia for cryoablation given their lower levels of associated pain during

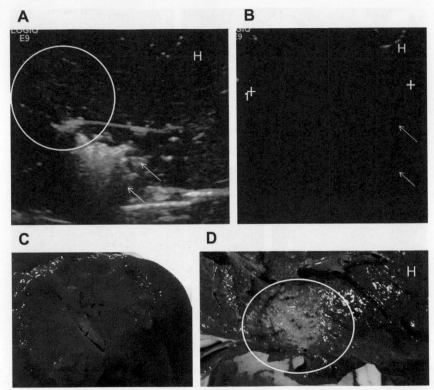

Fig. 6. Artifactual shadowing produced during RFA (*A*) and cryoablation (*B*) obscures the leading edge of the tumor with variable pathologic cryoablation (*C*) and RFA zones (*D*). Circle indicates probe (*A*) and ablation zone (*D*); arrows indicate shadowing artifact; calipers indicate estimated ablation zone diameter. H, liver.

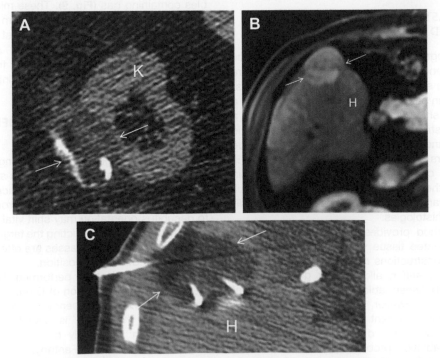

Fig. 7. CT clearly depicts the 0°C isotherm boundary in cryoablation of renal (*A*) and hepatic (*B, C*) masses. Arrows indicate lesion/cryoablation boundary. H, liver; K, kidney.

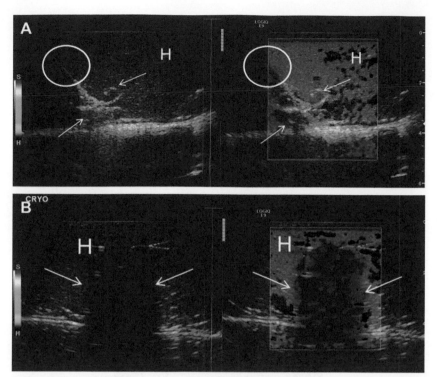

Fig. 8. Sonoelastography provides improved contrast of the ablation zone compared with B-mode US for RFA (*A*), but does not make a difference for cryoablation (*B*). Circle indicates probe; arrows indicate ablated tissue. H, liver.

treatment, while general anesthesia is often used for RFA at the authors' institution. Moderate sedation may be used during the RFA procedure, typically with greater doses of sedating agents.[27]

Topical anesthesia is created with 1% percutaneous lidocaine followed by probe placement under ultrasound guidance. If obstructing tissues are in the way or are limiting visualization of the probe tip, hydrodissection may be used (**Fig. 10**). Hydrodissection is the displacement of tissues by the injection of fluid, typically D5W, through a needle. A 22-gauge Chiba needle is advanced along the target plane with gradual injection of 50 to 100 mL of solution, creating a fluid barrier between adjacent structures and the probe. Artificial ascites do not prevent diaphragmatic injury when treating hepatic dome lesions.[28] An artificial pleural effusion can also be used to create a window between hepatic dome lesions and the lung in these cases, although this has been associated with pneumonia and respiratory dysfunction.[29]

Real-time monitoring of tine deployment is especially important in RFA to ensure that each tine has been fully extended and is not entering a vital structure such as the gallbladder, and adjacent bile ducts or vessels. Once the applicator has been successfully deployed, this process is repeated for additional probes.

The RFA procedure begins with placement of a grounding pad on the patient's skin, usually the thigh, to achieve a closed-loop circuit that will allow energy deposition to localize at the probe tip. Hair is stripped or shaved from the grounding pad location to avoid burns during the procedure.

The probes are then attached to the primary generator, and temperatures of 50°C to 100°C are maintained for 10 to 30 minutes to achieve in vivo cell death. Temperature sensors are present at the probe tips, which provide feedback for self-adjustment. Different probes measure cell death by different methods, such as levels of impedance (resistance to alternating current). As cell vaporization occurs, the resistance of tissue to the conduction of alternating currents increases. Once the impedance has "rolled off" or has significantly increased, the initial treatment cycle is complete. After a short interval (minutes), the process is repeated a varying number of times depending on the total ablation time and power wattage at roll-off. A cool-down cycle is then initiated, followed by retraction of the probe. Electrode tracts are coagulated on certain systems to maintain internal temperatures above 70°C.[4]

Cryoablation begins with the testing of a cryoprobe in a bowl of sterile water to assess ice-ball formation. The probe is then cooled and targeted to the lesion using US. Cryoprobes use tubing for

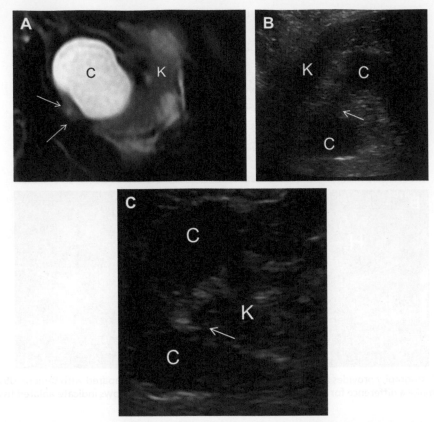

Fig. 9. A nodular component to a renal cyst is seen on one slice of an MR image (*A*) that is confirmed with contrast-enhanced US (*B*, *C*). The patient could not receive MRI or CT contrast because of renal dysfunction. Arrows indicate mural nodule. C, cyst; K, kidney.

the infusion of inert gas and thermocouples that are connected to the primary coolant machine. The machine is placed on stick mode, cooling the probes to at least −20°C over 2 separate intervals. The tissue is allowed to partially thaw at 5-minute to 8-minute intervals between cooling cycles, and the probes are then removed from the patient following a 5-minute thaw cycle after the

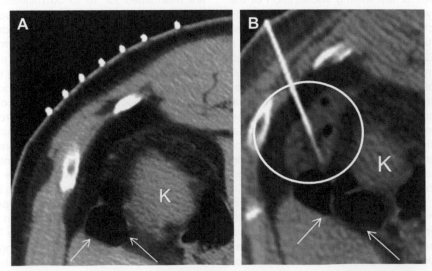

Fig. 10. Bowel lies near a renal lesion to be treated with ablation (*A*), and hydrodissection (*B*) is attempted to separate the bowel from tumor. Circle indicates D5W hydrodissection; arrows indicate bowel. K, kidney.

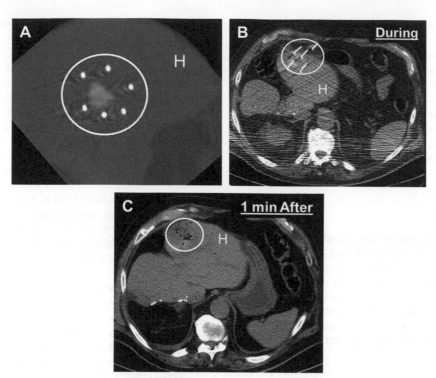

Fig. 11. Multiple tines are oriented geometrically (*A*) with subsequent IRE ablation of the tumor (*B*). Delayed imaging may show persistent gas in the ablation zone (*C*). Circle indicates tines and ablation zone. H, liver.

last cooling phase. Each cooling cycle lasts between 8 and 12 minutes.

Postprocedure imaging is then obtained to determine the area of treatment. RFA may be monitored with CEUS if there is no acoustic shadowing from gas formation. If gas is present, the imaging can be delayed for 60 minutes until the gas clears. In contrast, postprocedure cryoablation treatment zones are typically monitored with CT and MRI.

ALTERNATIVE METHODS OF ABLATION

IRE is a novel method of treatment using applied voltage gradients to alter membrane permeability and induce cell death. This process uses 1 or more probes placed at equally spaced intervals surrounding the tumor (**Fig. 11**). A small initial voltage is applied that induces transient permeability followed by an increase in voltage above a critical threshold that induces cell death.[30] IRE can be used to treat tumors near bile ducts and vessels, because the cell damage incurred on these structures is reversible and no heat-sink effect is observed. A large zone of edema surrounds the lesions initially, which clears within 24 hours (**Fig. 12**). Limitations of this treatment include vibration of the probes during ablation that can cause shear damage to surrounding

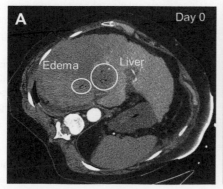
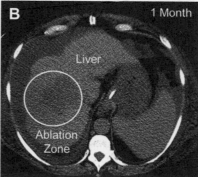

Fig. 12. Edema surrounds the liver immediately after treatment (*A*), extending well beyond the ablation zones (*circles*); this is better appreciated on delayed imaging (*B*).

tissue, and a systemic autoimmune response that is not well understood.

Microwave ablation produces thermal ablation by a mechanism similar to that of RFA, causing rapid vibration of water molecules. Advantages of this method are its rapid heating, broad lesion coverage, and lack of a significant heat sink.[31] Research regarding microwave ablation for the treatment of hepatocellular carcinoma is ongoing, but recent trials suggest an efficacy similar to that of RFA.

SUMMARY

US plays an important and increasing role in tumor ablation, especially in the liver and kidneys. Improvements in sonoelastography and CEUS allow for better tumor detection and monitoring before, after, and during the procedure. The use of US will likely continue to grow with these improvements, as it is readily accessible and affordable, provides real-time imaging, and is radiation free.

REFERENCES

1. Goldberg SN, Grassi CJ, Cardella JF, et al. Image-guided tumor ablation: standardization of terminology and reporting criteria. J Vasc Interv Radiol 2006;16:765–78.

2. Livraghi T, Festi D, Monti F, et al. US-guided percutaneous alcohol injection of small hepatic and abdominal tumors. Radiology 1986;161:309–12.

3. Hong K, Georgiades C. Radiofrequency ablation: mechanism of action and devices. J Vasc Interv Radiol 2010;8:S179–86.

4. Lencioni R, Crocetti L. Radiofrequency ablation of liver cancer. Tech Vasc Interv Radiol 2007;10:38–46.

5. Erinjeri JP, Clark TW. Cryoablation: mechanism of action and devices. J Vasc Interv Radiol 2001;12: 1020–32.

6. Maybody M, Solomon S. Image-guided percutaneous cryoablation of renal tumors. Tech Vasc Interv Radiol 2007;10:140–8.

7. Avadhani A, Tuite C, Sun W. Evaluation of the cancer patient. Interventional oncology principles. Cambridge (United Kingdom): Cambridge University Press; 2008. p. 23–7.

8. Lin S. Ultrasonography-guided radiofrequency ablation in hepatocellular carcinoma: current status and future perspectives. J Ultrasound Med 2013; 21:9–15.

9. Livarghi T. Guidelines for treatment of liver cancer. Eur J Ultrasound 2001;13:167–76.

10. McCarley JR, Soulen MC. Percutaneous ablation of hepatic tumors. Semin Intervent Radiol 2010;3: 255–60.

11. Gervais DA. Cryoablation versus radiofrequency ablation for renal tumor ablation: time to reassess? J Vasc Interv Radiol 2013;24:1135–8.

12. Gervias DA, McGovern FJ, Arellano RS, et al. Radiofrequency ablation of renal cell carcinoma. Part 1. Indications, results, and role in patient management over a 6-year period and ablation of 100 tumors. AJR Am J Roentgenol 2005;185:64–71.

13. Janzen NK, Perry KT, Han KR, et al. The effects of intentional cryoablation and radiofrequency ablation of renal tissue involving the collecting system in a porcine model. J Urol 2005;173:1368–74.

14. Kim PN, Choi D, Rhim H, et al. Planning ultrasound for percutaneous radiofrequency ablation to treat small (<3 cm) hepatocellular carcinomas detected on computed tomography or magnetic resonance imaging: a multicenter prospective study to assess factors affecting ultrasound visibility. J Vasc Interv Radiol 2012;23:627–34.

15. Lee MW, Lim HK, Kim YJ, et al. Percutaneous sonographically guided radiofrequency ablation of hepatocellular carcinoma. Causes of mistargeting and factors affecting the feasibility of a second ablation session. J Ultrasound Med 2011; 30:607–15.

16. Wood TF, Rose DM, Chung M, et al. Radiofrequency ablation of 231 unresectable hepatic tumors: indications, limitations and implications. Ann Surg Oncol 2000;7:593–600.

17. Lee MW, Rhim H, Cha DI, et al. Planning US for percutaneous radiofrequency ablation of small hepatocellular carcinomas (1-3cm): value of fusion imaging with conventional US and CT/MR images. J Vasc Interv Radiol 2013;24:958–65.

18. Goldberg SN, Dupuy DE. Image-guided radiofrequency tumor ablation: challenges and opportunities—part I. J Vasc Interv Radiol 2001;12:1020–32.

19. Rajesh S, Mukund A, Arora A, et al. Contrast-enhanced US-guided radiofrequency ablation of hepatocellular carcinoma. J Vasc Interv Radiol 2013; 24:1235–40.

20. Solbiati L, Goldberg SN, Ierace T, et al. Radiofrequency ablation of hepatic metastases: postprocedural assessment with a US microbubble contrast agent—early experience. Radiology 1999;211: 643–9.

21. Garra BS. Imaging and estimation of tissue elasticity by ultrasound. Ultrasound Q 2007;23:255–68.

22. Cho N, Moon WK, Kim HY, et al. Sonoelastographic strain index for differentiation of benign and malignant nonpalpable breast masses. J Ultrasound Med 2010;19:1–7.

23. Varghese T, Techavipoo U, Liu W, et al. Elastographic measurement of the area and volume of thermal lesions resulting from radiofrequency ablation: pathologic correlation. AJR Am J Roentgenol 2003;181:701–7.

24. Varghese T, Zagzebski JA, Lee FT. Elastographic imaging of thermal lesions in the liver in vivo following radiofrequency ablation: preliminary results. Ultrasound Med Biol 2002;28:1467–73.

25. Nielson MG. Contrast enhanced ultrasound. Eur J Radiol 2004;51(Suppl):S1.

26. Nielson MB, Bang N. Contrast enhanced ultrasound in liver imaging. Eur J Radiol 2004;51(Suppl):S3–8.

27. Truesdale CM, Soulen MC, Clark TW, et al. Percutaneous computed tomography-guided renal mass radiofrequency ablation versus cryoablation: doses of sedation medication used. J Vasc Interv Radiol 2013;24:347–50.

28. Kang TW, Rhim H, Lee MW, et al. Radiofrequency ablation for hepatocellular carcinoma abutting the diaphragm: comparison of effects of thermal protection and therapeutic efficacy. AJR Am J Roentgenol 2011;196:907–13.

29. Koda M, Ueki M, Maeda Y, et al. Percutaneous sonographically guided radiofrequency ablation with artificial pleural effusion for hepatocellular carcinoma located under the diaphragm. AJR Am J Roentgenol 2004;183:583–8.

30. Lee EW, Chen C, Prieto VE, et al. Advanced hepatic ablation technique for achieving complete cell death: irreversible electroporation. Radiology 2010; 255:426–33.

31. McWilliams JP, Yamamoto S, Raman SS, et al. Percutaneous ablation of hepatocellular carcinoma: current status. J Vasc Interv Radiol 2010;21:S204–13.

Ultrasound-Guided Biopsy of the Prostate: New Updates

Mehmet Ruhi Onur, MD[a], Ahmet Tuncay Turgut, MD[b],*,
Vikram Dogra, MD[c]

KEYWORDS

- Prostate • Transrectal ultrasonography • Biopsy

KEY POINTS

- To review the indications and contraindications for TRUS-guided biopsy of the prostate.
- To reveal the impact of various imaging tools on prostate biopsy technique.
- To discuss various methods of anesthesia used to relieve patient discomfort associated with the procedure.
- To discuss the impact of current updates on the technique and diagnostic accuracy of transrectal prostate biopsy.

DISCUSSION OF PROBLEM/CLINICAL PRESENTATION

Prostate cancer is the most frequently detected cancer in men, with about 700,000 patients diagnosed worldwide each year, accounting for 25% of new cancer cases in men and 9% of cancer-related deaths.[1,2] One in 6 men are affected by prostate cancer during their lifetime. Autopsy studies show foci of prostate cancer in up to 70% to 80% of 80-year-old men who died of other causes.[3] Prostate biopsy to diagnose prostate cancer with digital guidance was introduced by Astraldi in 1937.[4] The gold standard technique in the diagnosis of prostate cancer is transrectal ultrasound (TRUS)-guided biopsy, which was initially described by Wantanebe and colleagues in 1968.[5] Increased prostate-specific antigen (PSA) testing over the last 2 decades has resulted in increased prostate biopsies to show pathologic diagnosis of prostate cancer. Because the transrectal route is used in TRUS-guided prostate biopsy, this procedure has complication risks, mostly related to infection and bleeding. Although

TRUS-guided prostate biopsy is not a new technique, there has been increasing interest in providing appropriate prebiopsy preparation to prevent complications and increase the diagnostic accuracy of the technique in prostate cancer, with implementation of more accurate biopsy schemes and new imaging tools. In this article, new updates in TRUS-guided prostate biopsy are reviewed, including prebiopsy preparation, technique, complications, and recently implemented imaging tools such as contrast-enhanced ultrasonography, elastography, and magnetic resonance (MR) imaging–ultrasonography fused platforms to guide biopsy.

PREPROCEDURAL EVALUATION
Indications of TRUS-Guided Prostate Biopsy

A decision to perform a TRUS-guided prostate biopsy is mainly based on digital rectal examination (DRE) findings and PSA levels (**Box 1**). A suspicious DRE is an absolute indication for TRUS-guided prostate biopsy. Measurement of PSA levels has been the main screening test of prostate

[a] Department of Radiology, School of Medicine, University of Firat, Rektorluk Kampusu, Elazig 23119, Turkey;
[b] Department of Radiology, Ankara Training and Research Hospital, Ulucanlar Caddesi, Ankara 06590, Turkey;
[c] Department of Imaging Sciences, School of Medicine, University of Rochester, 601 Elmwood Avenue, Box 648, Rochester, NY 14642, USA
* Corresponding author.
E-mail address: ahmettuncayturgut@yahoo.com

Ultrasound Clin 9 (2014) 81–94
http://dx.doi.org/10.1016/j.cult.2013.09.002
1556-858X/14/$ – see front matter © 2014 Elsevier Inc. All rights reserved.

<table>
<tr><td>

Box 1
Indications for TRUS-guided prostate biopsy

Suspicious DRE findings

Increased levels of serum total PSA

PSA velocity greater than 0.75 ng/mL/y

Free PSA less than 20%, total PSA in gray zone

Ratio of pro-PSA to free PSA greater than 1.8%

Abnormal TRUS finding(s)

Before benign prostatic hyperplasia surgery

Evaluation for recurrence after failed radiation therapy before salvage local therapy

</td><td>

Box 2
Contraindications for prostate biopsy

Acute prostatitis

Urinary tract infections

Bleeding diathesis

Failure to take antibiotic prophylaxis

Intractable patient anxiety

Acute painful perianal disorders

</td></tr>
</table>

cancer. However, PSA is a nonspecific test, and using only PSA for the diagnosis may cause false-positive results for prostate cancer. PSA level may be increased in prostate cancer, benign prostatic hyperplasia (BPH), inflammation, after ejaculation, DRE, biopsy, and cystoscopy.[6] A PSA level of 4 ng/mL is accepted as an indication for prostate biopsy, although there is controversy around the threshold level for PSA.[6] The first test for increased PSA level should be repeated a few weeks later under the same conditions in the same laboratory using the same assay, before making a biopsy decision.[7,8] The cancer detection percentage of TRUS-guided prostate biopsy is 20% in patients with a PSA level greater than 2.5 ng/mL and 50% if the PSA level is greater than 10 ng/mL.[9] Indications of TRUS-guided prostate biopsy other than abnormal DRE and increased total PSA levels include PSA velocity greater than 0.75 ng/mL/y, free PSA less than 20%, total PSA in gray zone, ratio of pro-PSA to free PSA greater than 1.8%, abnormal TRUS finding(s), before BPH surgery, and evaluation for recurrence after failed radiation therapy before salvage local therapy. A PSA velocity of 0.75 ng/mL or greater per year is considered as suggestive of prostate cancer. In patients with PSA levels between 4 and 10 ng/mL, a cutoff value PSA density of 0.15 was also suggested to improve the detection rate of prostate cancer. Higher rate of cancer detection was noted in patients with free/total PSA of more than 15%.[10] Pro-PSA is more reliable than other forms of PSA in differentiating between cancer and benign conditions in men with PSA values from 2.5 to 10 ng/mL.

Among the main contraindications of prostate biopsy are acute prostatitis, urinary tract infections, bleeding diathesis, failure to take antibiotic prophylaxis, intractable patient anxiety, and acute painful perianal disorders (**Box 2**).

PATIENT DISCOMFORT AND ANESTHESIA
Patient Preparation

The steps to be followed during the preparation for TRUS-guided prostate biopsy include antibiotic prophylaxis, anticoagulant avoidance, and rectal cleansing with enema or laxative. It has been widely accepted that antibiotics and bowel preparation should be used to prevent the development of infection and sepsis after the procedure. Also, informing and reassuring the patient about the procedure are mandatory before biopsy.

Bowel cleansing
Prebiopsy bowel cleansing is recommended to visualize prostate adequately on TRUS and minimize infectious complications. Although some studies have shown that a cleansing enema is not required or recommended before biopsy,[11,12] it has been concluded in many others that a cleansing enema before biopsy may decrease bacteremia and bacteriuria after prostate biopsy.[13,14] Jeon and colleagues[15] reported that use of the prebiopsy rectal preparation was the most significant risk factor decreasing the development of infectious complications after the procedure. In that study, infectious complications developed in only 1.3% (6 of 456) of the patients who received the rectal preparation, whereas the relevant rate was 9.5% (40 of 423) among those who did not receive the preparation.[15] Some investigators concluded that administration of preventive antibiotics alone without rectal enema before prostate biopsy results in low infection rate, which may question the necessity of the rectal enema.[16] Carey and Korman[11] reported that clinically significant complications occurred in 4.4% of patients who had prebiopsy enemas and in 3.2% of patients who did not have prebiopsy enemas. It is suggested that rectal preparation could increase rectal irritation and might promote bacterial dissemination, resulting in increased infection risk.[17] Also, rectal enema increases patient cost and discomfort. In another

study, Ruddick and colleagues[18] found no significant difference between the rate of sepsis in patients who stopped eating by midnight on the day before the biopsy and had bowel cleansing. These conflicting results cause controversy about the necessity of prebiopsy rectal enema, and recent literature[11,12,18] suggests that prebiopsy rectal enemas were found to be ineffective in reducing infective complications.

Antibiotic prophylaxis
The use of antibiotic prophylaxis has been found to reduce the rates of infectious complications significantly. Antibiotic is administered before, the day of, and after TRUS. Broad-based gram-negative fluoroquinolones such as ciprofloxacin are most frequently used for antibiotic prophylaxis, with a global percentage of 92.5%.[19] Fluoroquinolones are well absorbed orally and have good prostate tissue levels.[20] A study[16] in which ciprofloxacin was used for prophylaxis with a dose of 500 mg twice daily for 8 doses beginning the day before the biopsy and continuing for 3 consecutive days resulted in approximately 0.1% infection rates. A single dose of fluoroquinolone was also reported to be as effective as multiple-dose prophylaxis.[21] Antibiotic prophylaxis has been switched or expanded because of increased fluoroquinolone resistance.[22] Almost 50% of postprostate biopsy-related infective symptoms were shown to be associated with fluoroquinolone-resistant organisms.[23] Gentamycin, metronidazole, amoxicillin-clavulanate, cefoxitin, trimethoprim-sulfamethoxazole, tosufloxacin, and ceftriaxone are recommended agents to switch or add to fluoroquinolons.[24]

Anticoagulant avoidance
Based on the fact that TRUS-guided biopsy has an inherent risk of hemorrhage, it is evident that measures should be taken to minimize the relevant risk, such as discontinuation of anticoagulant agents before the procedure. However, it is necessary to consult with hematologists in some clinical situations such as in patients with mechanical heart valves, atrial fibrillation with previous neurologic event, and recurrent or recent (<1 year ago) venous thromboembolism before discontinuation of anticoagulant agents.[25] The risk of hematuria was found to be increased 1.36-fold with aspirin usage in a meta-analysis including 3218 men.[26] Stopping aspirin in patients before prostate biopsy is unnecessary, unless an additional bleeding predisposition exists, because aspirin was not found to increase the risk of moderate and severe hematuria.[26] Coumadin (warfarin) is recommended to be stopped 5 days before biopsy after the

patient's coagulation is tested. Symptoms of infection should be monitored carefully in patients who use warfarin and antibiotics together because of the possible interaction of warfarin with various medications. Clopidogrel and ticlopidine should be stopped 7 to 10 days and 14 days, respectively, before the biopsy. Anticoagulant agents may be restarted within 24 hours of biopsy if no major bleeding occurs.[25]

Prebiopsy anesthesia
In general, the application of anesthesia is recommended during prostate biopsy, because patients usually feel discomfort and even pain during the procedure secondary to introduction and movement of the TRUS probe in the rectum and the needle piercing the rectum and the prostate capsule. The anesthesia techniques used in prostate biopsy include local (ie, intrarectal lubricant agents, periprostatic nerve blocks, caudal blocks, pudendal nerve blocks, and their different combinations) and systemic (ie, oral/intravenous drug administration and sedoanalgesia).[27]

Introduction of the probe into the rectum during prostate biopsy induces mechanical stretching of the sensory fibers located distal to the dentate line in the anal canal. Intrarectal lubricating agents provide satisfactory lubrication in order to reduce friction and protect the mucosa during probe insertion. The most frequently used lubricating agent is lidocaine, which is usually combined with prilocaine, nifedipine, dimethyl sulfoxide, and glyceryl trinitrate.[27] In a meta-analysis,[28] it was concluded that the effect size of these agents was not statistically significant, although intrarectal local anesthesia was reported to be associated with pain reduction compared with placebo.

The efficacy of periprostatic nerve block is well established in the literature, although optimal dosage and technique remain controversial. Periprostatic nerve block refers to injection of anesthetic drugs in to periprostatic nerves.[29] The most commonly used anesthetic agent is 5 to 10 mL of 1% or 2% injectable lidocaine without epinephrine, injected by a 22-gauge needle bilaterally at the site of the neurovascular bundle at the base of the gland just lateral to the junction between the prostate and seminal vesicles.[30] Although traditional periprostatic nerve block involves administration of lidocaine bilaterally, Taverna and colleagues[31] reported that a single injection of 10 mL of 1% lidocaine provides a similar efficiency of local anesthesia. Comparative studies with intrarectal lidocaine administration and periprostatic nerve block yielded more specific pain relief with the latter technique.[32] Alavi and colleagues[33] compared the pain scores of patients undergoing TRUS-guided prostate biopsy with the 2% lidocaine gel intrarectally or periprostatic infiltration with 1% aqueous lidocaine. The mean pain scores of the 2 groups were 3.7 versus 2.4 (P<.001) in favor of the infiltration group.

Periapical local anesthesia was also shown to provide significant pain relief though the combination of neurovascular bundle, and periapical local anesthesia was not reported to be superior to neurovascular bundle block alone for reducing pain during prostate biopsy.[34] A combination of intraglandular anesthesia and periprostatic nerve block provides more extensive coverage of sensory fibers and improves pain control compared with periprostatic nerve block only.[35] However, intraglandular lidocaine injections may cause vasovagal reactions.[36]

ANATOMY
Sonographic Anatomy

Thorough anatomic knowledge is essential for performing a successful TRUS-guided prostate biopsy. Technically, semicoronal, axial, and sagittal projections of the prostate can be obtained with end-viewing and side-viewing transducers. The hyperechoic peripheral zone is separated from the hypoechoic transitional zone by a hypoechoic line, representing the surgical capsule. Prostate cancer occurs most commonly in the peripheral zone (80%), followed by the transition zone (15%), and central zone (5%).[37] The sonographic appearance of the normal prostate varies depending on age. In young men, the hyperplasia of the glandular tissue is negligible, whereas in older men the development of BPH results in a larger gland with a more rounded shape.[38] Sonographically, the inner gland on the anterior aspect of the prostate has a hypoechoic appearance, whereas the outer peripheral zone is usually homogeneous and more echogenic. The relative amount of peripheral zone to inner gland increases from the base of the gland toward the apex.[39]

On TRUS, the anteriorly located hypoechoic transition zone can be discerned from the relatively echogenic peripheral zone, which is homogeneous in echotexture. The central zone, on the other hand, can hardly be differentiated from the peripheral zone on TRUS in healthy adult men. The transition zone constitutes an apparently larger proportion of the prostate in older men because of associated hyperplastic changes. Anatomically, the neurovascular bundles perforating the prostate capsule are critical, because they are a major site of capsular weakness and potentially prone to tumor involvement.[40]

IMAGING FEATURES

Adenocarcinomas constitute more than 95% of primary malignant prostate cancers. Transitional-cell carcinoma, sarcomas, and lymphoma are the other primary tumors of the prostate. Prostate cancer usually appears as a hypoechoic lesion on grayscale ultrasonography (**Fig. 1**). However, prostate cancers may manifest with an isoechoic or hyperechoic appearance secondary to desmoplastic response of the surrounding glandular tissue to the tumor, preexisting BPH, calcification, and uncommon histologic types of cancer.[41–43] Areas with asymmetrically increased and irregular flow on color flow Doppler ultrasonography (CDUS) or power Doppler ultrasonography (PDUS) refers to suspicious areas for prostate cancers (**Fig. 2**).[44] However, prostatitis, prostatic abscess, focal infection, and BPH nodules within the transition zone can manifest with increased flow on CDUS. The sensitivity of color Doppler TRUS for the diagnosis of prostate cancer ranges between 49% and 87%, and specificity ranges between 38% and 93%.[45,46] Because the gravity in the lateral decubitus position has been shown to affect position-related blood flow variation, CDUS or PDUS of the prostate should be performed when the patient is placed in the dorsal lithotomy position.[47]

BIOPSY PROTOCOLS
Technique of TRUS-Guided Prostate Biopsy

Patients lie in a left lateral decubitus position during the biopsy in order to avoid the collection of

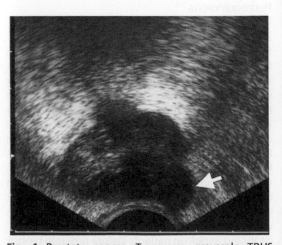

Fig. 1. Prostate cancer. Transverse grayscale TRUS image showing cancerous lesion with hypoechoic parenchymal echotexture and prominent posterior extracapsular extension of the cancerous tissue at the left peripheral zone (*arrow*) close to the rectal wall, implying infiltration.

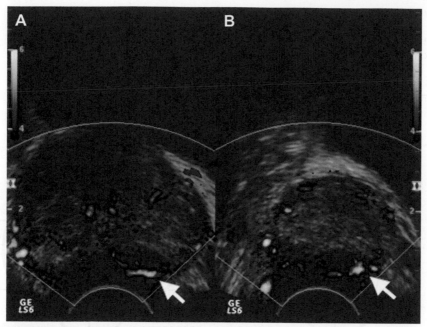

Fig. 2. Prostate cancer. Power Doppler TRUS images on transverse (*A*) and sagittal (*B*) planes showing hypoechoic lesion with asymmetrical vascularity (*arrows*) at the left paramedian aspect of the peripheral zone.

air in front of the ultrasound probe. Some physicians prefer the lithotomy position. Before probe insertion, a careful DRE should be undertaken in which tightness of the anal sphincter and presence of anal diseases such as anal fissures and rectal tumors should be investigated in order to avoid painful procedures and significant hemorrhage. Technically, circumferential examination of the rectum should be followed by digital examination of the prostate, which includes examination of the symmetry, size, and presence of nodules, tenderness, or pain in the prostate gland.

The initial step of grayscale ultrasonography should be identification of the transition zone, urethra, and peripheral zone of the prostate. Technically, transducers in the 5-MHz to 8-MHz range provide an optimal resolution for the peripheral zone, which might have a positive impact on the accuracy of the biopsy procedure. The volume of the prostate can be calculated with the ellipsoid formula by using the diameters in the orthogonal axes calculated on TRUS:

$$\text{Volume of prostate} = 0.52 \times \text{td} \times \text{apd} \times \text{ccd}$$

where td, apd, and ccd represent the transverse, anteroposterior, and craniocaudal diameters of the prostate, respectively.

After the measurement of the prostate size, prostate nodules, which are typically hypoechoic, should be notified, followed by assessment of the rectal wall, prostate capsule, and seminal

vesicles. Biopsy specimens may be obtained with 18-gauge needles using an automated biopsy gun (**Fig. 3**). To avoid contamination with the periprostatic tissue and to enable extraction of a longer tissue sample, the sampling procedure should be performed after indenting the prostate capsule with the biopsy needle.[48] Classically, sextant sampling sites are the cores at the midway between the lateral border and the median plane at the levels of the base, midgland, and apex of the prostate, respectively (**Fig. 4**). Extended biopsy protocol, on the other hand, involves the sampling of laterally directed cores.

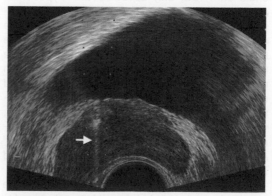

Fig. 3. Transverse grayscale TRUS image depicting the trajectory of the needle (*arrow*) used for sampling medial aspect of the prostate at the level of midgland.

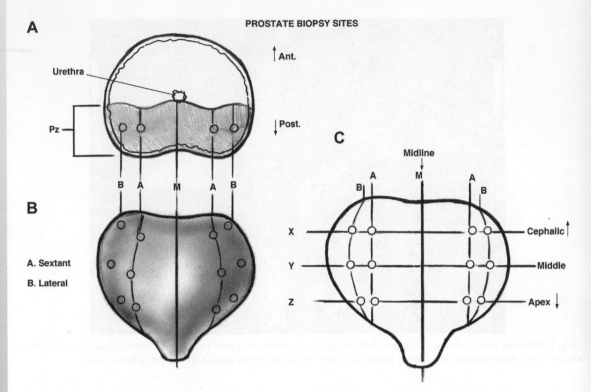

PROSTATE BIOPSY SITES

Fig. 4. Axial (*A*), posteroanterior (PA) (*B*), and coronal (*C*) views of the prostate showing the anatomic localizations of the biopsy cores in sextant (*A*) and lateral (*B*) sampling protocols. In the extended sampling protocol, additional cores lateral to the sites for the classical sextant biopsy at the base (*X*), middle part (*Y*), and apex (*Z*) of the prostate are targeted. Ant., anterior; Post., posterior; Pz, peripheral zone. (*From* Turgut AT, Dogra VS. Transrectal prostate biopsies. In: Dogra V, Saad W, editors. Ultrasound guided procedures. 1st ed. New York: Thieme; 2009. p. 90; with permission.)

Systematic biopsy

Taking into account that approximately 50% of prostate cancers are not visible on conventional grayscale TRUS, the sampling of the prostate gland should be performed systematically.[6,49] Although prostate cancers usually appear hypoechoic on TRUS, only about 50% of hypoechoic areas in prostate are cancerous tissue.[50] Nonvisualized prostate cancers are usually low-grade cancers. Most prostate cancers are infiltrative rather than a well-defined mass (**Fig. 5**). More than 30% of prostate cancers are isoechoic, which makes them nonvisible on ultrasonography and necessitates systematic biopsies. Isoechoic tumors may be targeted in systematic biopsies, with the imaging findings consisting of gland asymmetry, capsular bulge, and posterior attenuation.[43] Anatomically, prostate cancers are mostly located in the apex and base of the peripheral gland.

In systematic biopsy, typically, 12 samples are obtained, accompanied by additional samples from any suspicious areas seen on TRUS.[6] Autopsy studies have shown sextant prostate biopsy sensitivities at 30%, with increasing sensitivity with

increasing numbers of biopsy cores: 36% to 58% for 12-core biopsies and 53% to 58% for 18-core biopsies.[51] If the patient does not tolerate the procedure at the beginning, suspicious areas should

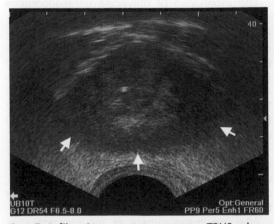

Fig. 5. Infiltrative prostate cancer. TRUS shows prostate cancer in infiltrative pattern (*arrows*) with hypoechoic appearance through peripheral zone of prostate.

be sampled first. Mathematically, increasing the number of cores results in increased sensitivity for detection of prostate cancer. However, the direction of the biopsies is as important as the number of the cores. In this regard, laterally directed sextant biopsy enables sampling of the far-lateral midlobar region, where most of the extra cancers are detected (see **Fig. 4**).[52]

The negative predictive value of a systematic TRUS-guided biopsy was reported in the range of 36% to 89%.[53] Also, systematic biopsies underestimate the true Gleason score calculated on prostatectomy specimens.

Targeted biopsy

Targeted biopsy of the prostate refers to sampling of any area of the prostate that is localized by advanced imaging modalities such as CDUS or PDUS, contrast-enhanced ultrasonography, ultrasonographic elastography, or MR imaging–ultrasonography fusion. Recent advances in multiparametric MR imaging and the development of novel ultrasonographic techniques, such as contrast-enhanced ultrasonography and elastography, may favor targeted biopsies, enabling the sampling of fewer cores compared with systematic biopsy. Classically, hypoechoic areas in the prostate on grayscale ultrasonography are the main targets during prostate biopsies. The positive predictive value of the biopsy of a peripheral hypoechoic lesion for prostate cancer is 25% to 30%.[42] Color Doppler imaging shows areas of increased vascularity, which may be associated with tumor sites. Target lesions in prostate present with decreased elasticity on elasticity imaging.

Comparison between contrast-enhanced harmonic imaging–targeted biopsy versus systematic biopsy revealed that targeted biopsy was 1.5 times more likely to find cancer than was systematic biopsy.[54] However, targeted biopsies may miss 20% of cancers, which were detected only on systematic biopsy alone, leading to the conclusion that targeted biopsies cannot replace systematic biopsies, according to current literature.[55]

Follow-up TRUS-guided prostate biopsy

Follow-up TRUS-guided biopsy is performed when initial biopsy results are negative although high clinical suspicion remains for prostate cancer or initial biopsy yielded atypical small acinar proliferation or high-grade prostate intraepithelial neoplasia (HGPIN). Follow-up biopsy includes 12 to 17 samples from the prostate parenchyma in a systematic fashion. Cancer detection rates increase by 5% to 35% with follow-up biopsy as opposed to initial systematic biopsies.[52,56,57] The transition zone of the prostate should be sampled

at repeat biopsy, although it is not recommended at initial biopsy.

Proper management of patients with HGPIN is not yet established. The detection rate of prostate cancer in men who had the diagnosis of HGPIN in previous biopsy is the same with the risk of cancer on a repeat biopsy if the initial biopsy results are negative.[58] Extended prostate biopsy with 12 cores does not seem to necessitate repeat biopsy in the setting of HGPIN if the biopsy technique is adequate. However, repeat biopsy is indicated in patients with results of atypical glands that were suspicious but not diagnostic of cancer in previous biopsy.[52]

Saturation biopsy

Saturation biopsy refers to acquisition of more than 20 core biopsies from prostate parenchyma in a systematic manner. Although saturation biopsy shows more accurate results than 12-core systematic biopsy in detection of prostate cancer, because of increased number of biopsy cores, this technique should be reserved for repeat biopsy in the setting of negative results on initial biopsy with suspicion of prostate cancer. The rate of detection of prostate cancer on saturation biopsies is 29% to 41% in patients with a suspicion for cancer and previous negative biopsies.[59–61] Even saturation biopsies may miss significant cancers.[62] A transperineal approach may be used as an alternative, although the technique has a 2-fold risk for complications compared with 12-core to 18-core techniques.[63,64]

Transperineal biopsy

Transperineal biopsy with ultrasound guidance can be used to obtain tissue diagnosis in prostate cancer in patients with a closed anal orifice after previous surgery for rectal cancer. It is safe to perform transperineal biopsy without routine antibiotic prophylaxis.[65] Detection rates of prostate cancer of transperineal and transrectal prostate biopsies were not found to be significantly different when the same number of cores was used.[66,67] Intravenous sedation is preferred to provide analgesia. Transperineal prostate biopsy can be performed when the patient is in the lithotomy position. Biopsy of the prostate starts after cleaning the perineum with 5% chlorhexidine solution, draping the scrotum anteriorly to access the perineum, and infiltration of local anesthetic in the perineal skin and subcutaneous tissue.[65] An eighteen-gauge biopsy needle is used for sampling in transperineal biopsy of the prostate.

In several studies with more patients, about 1 of 5 prostate cancers have been shown to be located in the anterior region of the prostate.[68,69] A transperineal biopsy approach provides easy access to these regions of the prostate gland, and several investigators have reported a higher rate of prostate cancer found using this approach.[70,71] The results of a meta-analysis showed that there was no difference for cancer detection rate between the extensive transrectal and transperineal group, as well as between the saturation transrectal and transperineal approaches.[72] Also, no significant differences were found between the 2 approaches for the incidence of major or minor complications.[72]

Advanced Imaging Techniques

Advanced imaging techniques in TRUS-guided biopsy include contrast-enhanced ultrasonography, ultrasound elastography, and MR imaging–ultrasonography fusion, which are used in targeted biopsy of the prostate. These imaging techniques are mainly used to detect prostate cancers that are nonvisible on grayscale ultrasonography and as a guide to biopsy the detected lesions. Prostate cancers located in the far anterior prostate and transitional zones may be difficult to detect by conventional TRUS. Contrast-enhanced ultrasonography and elastography may be used as complementary techniques in detection of these lesions.

Transrectal contrast-enhanced ultrasound-guided biopsy

Contrast-enhanced ultrasonography depicts microneovascularity in prostate cancer more accurately than CDUS or PDUS.[73] Contrast-enhanced TRUS-guided biopsy studies yielded higher sensitivity of detecting cancer than unenhanced ultrasonography.[74] However, the specificity of contrast-enhanced and unenhanced ultrasonography was not significantly different.[75] Halpern and colleagues[54] reported significantly improved sensitivity, from 38% to 65%, for detecting prostate cancer, with preserved specificity at approximately 80%. Addition of contrast-enhanced ultrasonography to unenhanced ultrasonographic imaging improves detection rates of prostate cancer. Premedication with dutasteride (a dual 5-α reductase inhibitor) for 7 to 14 days before biopsy can improve detection of cancer with contrast-enhanced ultrasonography, by reducing prostatic blood flow in benign prostatic tissue and making cancerous tissue more visible.[76] A suspicious site on contrast-enhanced ultrasonography was found to be 5 times more likely to have a positive finding on prostate biopsy than a standard sextant site.[77] Targeted biopsy with contrast-enhanced Doppler ultrasonography has an advantage over systematic biopsy, with detection of several tumors equal to that of systematic biopsies with fewer than half the cores.[78]

Elastography

Prostate cancer presents with increased stiffness and decreased elasticity on ultrasound elastography. The viscosity parameter of prostate cancer was shown to be 2.4 times greater than normal tissue.[79] Areas of decreased elasticity were found to be more than twice as likely to be malignant compared with areas with normal elasticity.[49] The detection rate of prostate cancer for biopsy cores was found to be significantly better in the elastography-targeted cores (12.7%) than in the systematic biopsies (5.6%).[80]

Konig and colleagues[81] reported a high sensitivity rate of ultrasound elastography of 84.1% compared with 64.2% using grayscale TRUS in detection of prostate cancer. A sonoelastographic study including 492 patients found the sensitivity, specificity, and negative predictive values in the diagnosis of prostate cancer to be 86%, 72%, and 91.4%.[82] Positive ultrasound elastographic findings were found to be associated more with the increase in Gleason scores than the CDUS findings.[49]

MR IMAGING–ASSISTED BIOPSIES

Multiparametric MR imaging of the prostate refers to assessment of prostate with combination of T2-weighted imaging, diffusion-weighted imaging, and perfusion-weighted imaging. Multiparametric MR imaging is helpful for imaging guided biopsy techniques by its localizing strength. TRUS-guided biopsies may be performed more accurately with the images created from fusion of previously acquired MR imaging data and real-time ultrasonographic images. In MR imaging–TRUS-guided biopsy, samples are obtained from lesions suspicious for prostate cancer that were identified on prebiopsy MR imaging (**Figs. 6** and **7**). Targeted biopsy by fusing MR imaging and ultrasonography may be performed with 2 methods: fusion of MR imaging and ultrasonographic images on a platform, including ultrasound equipment and electromagnetic tracking or mechanical-arm navigation and cognitive fusion of MR imaging and ultrasonographic images. MR imaging–TRUS fusion can map the lesion and location of all the obtained cores.[83]

MR imaging–TRUS fusion-guided biopsy starts with a two-dimensional TRUS sweep of the prostate in the axial plane to render a three-dimensional ultrasonographic image, followed by fusion of three-dimensional ultrasonographic images with prebiopsy MR imaging. In this way, suspected lesions for prostate cancer on MR imaging can be superimposed on ultrasonographic

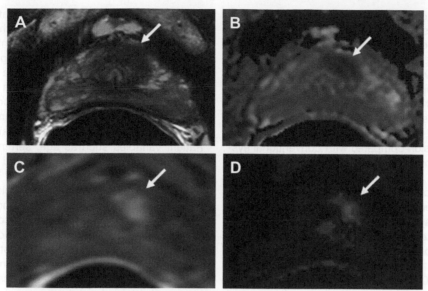

Fig. 6. MR imaging–TRUS fusion-guided prostate biopsy. A 66-year-old man with serum PSA of 10.10 ng/mL with 2 previous negative TRUS-guided biopsies. (*A*) Axial T2-weighted MR imaging, (*B*) apparent diffusion coefficient map of diffusion-weighted image, (*C*) raw dynamic contrast-enhanced MR imaging, and (*D*) Ktrans map derived from dynamic contrast-enhanced MR imaging show a left apical anterior transitional zone lesion (*arrow*). Subsequent transrectal ultrasonography/MR imaging fusion-guided biopsies showed Gleason 4 + 4 cancer in the lesion (80% core involvement). (*Courtesy of* Barış Turkbey, MD, National Cancer Institute, National Institutes of Health, Bethesda, MD.)

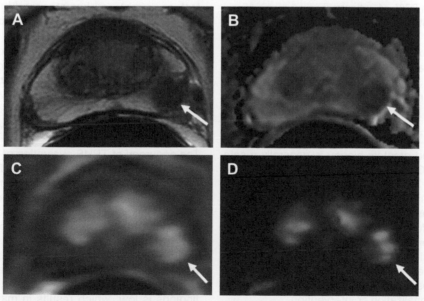

Fig. 7. MR imaging–TRUS fusion-guided prostate biopsy. A 58-year-old man with serum PSA of 4.7 ng/mL with 2 previous TRUS-guided biopsies with a result of Gleason 3 + 3 cancer on the left with less than 5% of core involvement. (*A*) Axial T-weighted MR imaging, (*B*) apparent diffusion coefficient map of diffusion-weighted image, (*C*) raw dynamic contrast-enhanced MR imaging, and (*D*) Ktrans map derived from dynamic contrast-enhanced MR imaging show a left midperipheral zone lesion (*arrow*). Subsequent transrectal ultrasonography/MR imaging fusion-guided biopsies showed Gleason 4 + 4 cancer in the lesion (90% core involvement). (*Courtesy of* Barış Turkbey, MD, National Cancer Institute, National Institutes of Health, Bethesda, MD.)

images. Tracking of the direction of the biopsy needle and sampling the lesion can be visualized on a three-dimensional reconstructed image of the prostate.[84]

In cognitive fusion, the ultrasound operator directs the biopsy needle at the prostate area where the previous MR imaging has shown a lesion. A review of 22 studies[85] concluded improved accuracy in the diagnosis of prostate cancer with cognitive fusion compared with conventional systematic biopsy.

Pinto and colleagues[84] reported higher cancer detection per core with MR imaging–TRUS fusion-guided biopsy than standard 12-core TRUS biopsy. In their study, these investigators classified the lesions as low, moderate, and high suspicion for cancer on MR imaging and found that cancer was detected in 23 of 158 (14.6%), 29 of 72 (40.3%), and 24 of 34 (70.6%) lesions with low-suspicion, moderate-suspicion, and high-suspicion groups.[84] Marks and colleagues[86] reported that targeted biopsies with MR imaging–TRUS fusion were 2 to 3 times more sensitive for detection of prostate cancer than nontargeted systematic biopsies in more than 600 patients. Siddiqui and colleagues[83] compared the Gleason scores of biopsy specimens obtained by MR imaging–TRUS fusion-guided prostate biopsy with a standard 12-core biopsy regimen alone. In their study, addition of targeted biopsy led to Gleason upgrading in 32% of patients.

Major limitations of MR imaging–TRUS fusion are patient movement, time-consuming motion compensation, and gland swelling after the initial biopsies, leading to misregistration.[6] Also, this technique is indirect, involves use of an additional device, and requires specialized operator training.

Complications of TRUS-Guided Biopsy

TRUS-guided prostate biopsy is generally a safe procedure. Complications of TRUS-guided prostate biopsy include hematuria, hematospermia, rectal bleeding, infection, lower urinary tract symptoms, dysuria, epididymitis, urinary retention, erectile dysfunction, and mortality. Minor complications after prostate biopsy occur in 64% to 78% of patients.[87] Major complications include sepsis, severe rectal bleeding and hematuria, prostate abscess, and urinary retention, which require hospitalization or intervention.

Hypotensive vasovagal reactions may occur during or after the biopsy in 1% to 6% of patients after prostate biopsy, which necessitates observing patients for about an hour after biopsy.[88] Vasovagal reactions occurring after prostate biopsy usually recover spontaneously.

The most important complications after prostate biopsy are infection and sepsis, which may cause hospitalization. In the absence of antibiotic prophylaxis, bacteriuria occurs in 8% of patients after TRUS-guided prostate biopsy, with a clinical rate of urinary tract infection of 5% and a hospitalization rate of 2%.[89] Number of biopsy cores was reported to be one of the most significant factors for infectious complications after prostate biopsy.[15] Patient variables such as age, serum PSA level, and prostate volume are not related to the incidence of infectious complications.[15] There are some patient groups that alert clinicians to be more careful about sepsis occurrence. Patients on steroid medication or immunocompromised patients have a tendency for infection and may require a longer course of antibiotics. Biopsy should be avoided during urinary infection and for 4 to 6 weeks thereafter. Duplessis and colleagues[90] obtained rectal cultures before TRUS biopsy and used antimicrobial susceptibility results to develop an antibiotic prophylaxis regimen. These investigators observed no infectious complications after biopsy and concluded that rectal cultures obtained before TRUS biopsy, using selective media to identify fluoroquinolone-resistant Enterobacteriaceae, facilitate targeted antibiotic prophylaxis, and seem to be highly efficacious in reducing infectious complications.

Bleeding after TRUS-guided biopsy may manifest as hematuria, hematospermia, and hematochezia which are usually self-limiting. Minor bleeding may be observed in the urine, stool, and in the ejaculate after prostate biopsy. Generally, blood in the urine, stool, and ejaculate disappears in few days, although discolored semen may last for 6 to 8 weeks.[6]

PEARLS, PITFALLS, AND VARIANTS

The accuracy of TRUS evaluation of the prostate gland for cancer is not satisfactory. Evaluation of the prostate by TRUS can be complicated by BPH in the elderly population. Although TRUS-guided biopsy with 12 cores is accepted as the gold standard for the diagnosis of prostate cancer in most centers, imaging data obtained by TRUS cannot obviate systematic sampling of the gland. The positive predictive value of prostate biopsies based on DRE, PSA, and TRUS findings is low, which results in many unnecessary biopsies.

PATHOLOGY

The pathology results for most patients are usually straightforward and definitive in patients with prostate cancer. However, a significant controversy exists for the management of patients with HGPIN, whose biopsy specimens may infrequently show atypical cells during pathologic analysis. Mostly, the diagnosis of HGPIN after initial prostate biopsy is regarded to be either precancerous or concurrent with cancer in a remote location. Therefore, a repeat prostate biopsy is recommended for patients with the relevant histopathology, because they are considered to have increased malignancy risk.[40] A repeat biopsy in these patients should involve sampling of the whole gland, including the inner gland and high predilection areas of the peripheral zone rather than focusing on the sites with HGPIN reported in the initial biopsy.[38]

The small tumor volume or inappropriate sampling by the needle passing through the edge of an adjacent tumor may result in nondiagnostic cellular changes histopathologically. Accordingly, a site-specific approach focusing around the suspicious areas is recommended in these patients.

Measurement of the tumor aggressiveness in prostate cancer can be performed with Gleason grade, referring to the numerical encoding of the relevant assessment of histopathologic analysis of biopsy specimen. In this regard, the Gleason grading system combines discrete primary and secondary patterns or grades into a total of 9 discrete groups (scores 2–10). Accordingly, the primary grade refers to the predominant grade, with the secondary grade representing the next most common one. A Gleason score less than 4 is consistent with a well-differentiated cancer, whereas one greater than 7 represents poorly differentiated, aggressive tumors. Apart from the Gleason score, the number of cores harboring the diseased cells and the percentage of tumor in each core are other factors that should be taken into consideration for the management of the tumor and the assessment of the prognosis.

WHAT THE REFERRING PHYSICIAN NEEDS TO KNOW

Awareness of the advantages and limitations of TRUS-guided biopsy technique, as well as recent advances, is critical, because this enables the physician to avoid any mismanagement during the course of the disease. In general, it is agreed that TRUS-guided biopsy of the prostate is the gold standard method for the diagnosis of prostate cancer. The procedure is generally safe and well tolerated, although it may frequently be accompanied by minor complications.

SUMMARY

The diagnosis of prostate cancer depends on histopathologic confirmation. TRUS-guided biopsy of the prostate is the gold standard for the detection of prostate cancer. Decreasing complications of TRUS-guided prostate biopsy such as infection and bleeding and increasing patient comfort by providing adequate anesthesia has been the main purpose of studies regarding prebiopsy preparation of patient. Targeted and saturation biopsy schemes have improved detection rates for prostate cancer over standard systematic biopsy schemes but carry additional morbidity and cost and do not seem to replace the systematic 12-core biopsy in the diagnosis of prostate cancer. Advances in multiparametric MR imaging, contrast-enhanced ultrasonography, and elastography may result in use of these techniques as complementary methods, with the advantages of decreased biopsy attempts and complications.

REFERENCES

1. Parkin DM, Bray F, Ferlay J, et al. Global cancer statistics, 2002. CA Cancer J Clin 2005;55:74–108.
2. Jemal A, Siegel R, Ward E, et al. Cancer statistics, 2009. CA Cancer J Clin 2009;59:225–49.
3. Breslow N, Chan CW, Dhom G, et al. Latent carcinoma of prostate at autopsy in seven areas. The International Agency for Research on Cancer, Lyon, France. Int J Cancer 1977;20(5):680–8.
4. Astraldi A. Diagnosis of cancer of the prostate: biopsy by rectal route. Urol Cutaneous Rev 1937;41:421–2.
5. Wantanabe H, Kato H, Kato T, et al. Diagnostic application of the ultrasonotomography for the prostate. Nihon Hinyokika Gakkai Zasshi 1968;59:273–9.
6. Ghai S, Toi A. Role of transrectal ultrasonography in prostate cancer. Radiol Clin North Am 2012;50:1061–73.
7. Eastham JA, Riedel E, Scardino PT, et al, Polyp Prevention Trial Study Group. Variation of serum prostate-specific antigen levels: an evaluation of year-to-year fluctuations. JAMA 2003;289(20):2695–700.
8. Stephan C, Klaas M, Muller C, et al. Interchangeability of measurements of total and free prostate-specific antigen in serum with 5 frequently used assay combinations: an update. Clin Chem 2006;52(1):59–64.
9. Toi A, Neill MG, Lockwood GA, et al. The continuing importance of transrectal ultrasound identification of prostatic lesions. J Urol 2007;177:516–20.
10. Pelzer AE, Volgger H, Bektic J, et al. The effect of percentage free prostate-specific antigen (PSA)

level on the prostate cancer detection rate in a screening population with low PSA levels. BJU Int 2005;96:995–8.

11. Carey JM, Korman HJ. Transrectal ultrasound guided biopsy of the prostate. Do enemas decrease clinically significant complications? J Urol 2001;166:82–5.

12. Kang MY, Park JH, Kwak C, et al. Transrectal needle biopsy of the prostate: the efficacy of a pre-biopsy enema. Korean J Urol 2008;49:248–51.

13. Kim SJ, Kim SI, Ahn HS, et al. Risk factors for acute prostatitis after transrectal biopsy of the prostate. Korean J Urol 2010;51(6):426–30.

14. Lindert KA, Kabalin JN, Terris MK. Bacteremia and bacteriuria after transrectal ultrasound guided prostate biopsy. J Urol 2000;164:76–80.

15. Jeon SS, Woo SH, Hyun JH, et al. Bisacodyl rectal preparation can decrease infectious complications of transrectal ultrasound-guided prostate biopsy. Urology 2003;62(3):461–6.

16. Sieber PR, Rommel FM, Agusta VE, et al. Antibiotic prophylaxis in ultrasound guided transrectal prostate biopsy. J Urol 1997;157:2199–200.

17. Vallancien G, Prapotnich D, Veillon B, et al. Systemic prostatic biopsies in 100 men with no suspicion of cancer on digital rectal examination. J Urol 1991;146:1308–12.

18. Ruddick F, Sanders P, Bicknell SG, et al. Sepsis rates after ultrasound-guided prostate biopsy using a bowel preparation protocol in a community hospital. J Ultrasound Med 2011;30(2):213–6.

19. Wagenlehner FM, van Oostrum E, Tenke P, et al. Infective complications after prostate biopsy: outcome of the Global Prevalence Study of Infections in Urology (GPIU) 2010 and 2011, a prospective multinational multicentre prostate biopsy study. Eur Urol 2013;63(3):521–7.

20. Hori S, Sengupta A, Joannides A, et al. Changing antibiotic prophylaxis for transrectal ultrasound-guided prostate biopsies: are we putting our patients at risk? BJU Int 2010;106(9):1298–302.

21. Aron M, Rajeev TP, Gupta NP. Antibiotic prophylaxis for transrectal needle biopsy of the prostate: a randomized controlled study. BJU Int 2000; 85(6):682–5.

22. Bootsma AM, Laguna Pes MP, Geerlings SE, et al. Antibiotic prophylaxis in urologic procedures: a systematic review. Eur Urol 2008;54(6):1270–86.

23. Ongün S, Aslan G, Avkan-Oguz V. The effectiveness of single-dose fosfomycin as antimicrobial prophylaxis for patients undergoing transrectal ultrasound-guided biopsy of the prostate. Urol Int 2012;89(4):439–44.

24. Loeb S, Vellekoop A, Ahmed HU, et al. Systematic review of complications of prostate biopsy. Eur Urol 2013. http://dx.doi.org/10.1016/j.eururo.2013.05.049.

25. Kearon C, Hirsh J. Management of anticoagulation before and after elective surgery. N Engl J Med 1997;336:1506–11.

26. Carmignani L, Picozzi S, Bozzini G, et al. Transrectal ultrasound-guided prostate biopsies in patients taking aspirin for cardiovascular disease: a meta-analysis. Transfus Apher Sci 2011;45(3):275–80.

27. Maccagnano C, Scattoni V, Roscigno M, et al. Anaesthesia in transrectal prostate biopsy: which is the most effective technique? Urol Int 2011; 87(1):1–13.

28. Tiong HY, Liew LC, Samuel M, et al. A metaanalysis of local anesthesia for transrectal ultrasound-guided biopsy of the prostate. Prostate Cancer Prostatic Dis 2007;10:127–36.

29. Turgut AT, Ergun E, Koşar U, et al. Sedation as an alternative method to lessen patient discomfort due to transrectal ultrasonography-guided prostate biopsy. Eur J Radiol 2006;57:148–53.

30. Nash PA, Bruce JE, Indudhara R, et al. Transrectal ultrasound guided prostatic nerve blockade eases systematic needle biopsy of the prostate. J Urol 1996;155:607–9.

31. Taverna G, Maffezzini M, Benetti A, et al. A single injection of lidocaine as local anesthesia for ultrasound guided needle biopsy of the prostate. J Urol 2002;167:222–3.

32. Stirling BN, Shockley KF, Carothers GG, et al. Comparison of local anesthesia techniques during transrectal ultrasound-guided biopsies. Urology 2002;60:89–92.

33. Alavi AS, Soloway MS, Vaidya A, et al. Local anesthesia for ultrasound guided prostate biopsy: a prospective randomized trial comparing 2 methods. J Urol 2001;166:1343–5.

34. Cevik I, Dillioglugil O, Zisman A, et al. Combined "periprostatic and periapical" local anesthesia is not superior to "periprostatic" anesthesia alone in reducing pain during Tru-Cut prostate biopsy. Urology 2006;68:1215–9.

35. Cam K, Sener M, Kayikci A, et al. Combined periprostatic and intraprostatic local anesthesia for prostate biopsy: a double-blind, placebo controlled, randomized trial. J Urol 2008;180: 141–4.

36. Turgut AT, Ölçücüoglu E, Kosar P, et al. Complications and limitations related to periprostatic local anesthesia before TRUS-guided prostate biopsy. J Clin Ultrasound 2008;36:67–71.

37. Sexton WJ, Spiess PE, Pisters LL, et al. Are there differences in zonal distribution and tumor volume of prostate cancer in patients with a positive family history? Int Braz J Urol 2010;36(5):571–82.

38. Turgut AT, Dogra VS. Prostate carcinoma: evaluation using transrectal sonography. In: Hayat MA, editor. Methods of cancer diagnosis, therapy and

prognosis. 1st edition. New York: Elsevier; 2008. p. 499–520.

39. Turgut AT, Dogra VS, MacLennan G. Neoplasms of the prostate and seminal vesicles. In: Dogra VS, Maclennan GT, editors. Genitourinary radiology: the pathologic basis. London: Springer-Verlag; 2013. p. 45–71.

40. Turgut AT, Kısmalı E, Dogra V. Ultrasound of the prostate: update on current techniques. Ultrasound Clin 2010;5(3):475–8.

41. Dahnert WF, Hamper UM, Walsh PC, et al. The echogenic focus in prostatic sonograms, with xe-roradiographic and histopathologic correlation. Radiology 1986;159:95–100.

42. Rifkin MD, Dahnert W, Kurtz AB. State of the art: endorectal sonography of the prostate gland. AJR Am J Roentgenol 1990;154:691–700.

43. Hamper UM, Sheth S, Walsh PC, et al. Bright echogenic foci in early prostatic carcinoma: sonographic and pathologic correlation. Radiology 1990;176:339–43.

44. Turgut AT, Olçücüoglu E, Koşar P, et al. Power Doppler ultrasonography of the feeding arteries of the prostate gland: a novel approach to the diagnosis of prostate cancer? J Ultrasound Med 2007; 26:875–83.

45. Amiel GE, Slawin KM. Newer modalities of ultrasound imaging and treatment of the prostate. Urol Clin North Am 2006;33:329–37.

46. Pallwein L, Mitterberger M, Gradl J, et al. Value of contrast-enhanced ultrasound and elastography in imaging of prostate cancer. Curr Opin Urol 2007;17:39–47.

47. Halpern EJ, Frauscher F, Forsberg F, et al. High-frequency Doppler US of the prostate: effect of patient position. Radiology 2002;222:634–9.

48. Papatheodorou A, Ellinas P, Tandeles S, et al. Transrectal ultrasonography and ultrasound-guided biopsies of the prostate gland: how, when, and where. Curr Probl Diagn Radiol 2005;34:76–83.

49. Nelson ED, Slotoroff CB, Gomella LG, et al. Targeted biopsy of the prostate: the impact of color Doppler imaging and elastography on prostate cancer detection and Gleason score. Urology 2007;70(6):1136–40.

50. Dyke CH, Toi A, Sweet JM. Value of random ultrasound-guided transrectal prostate biopsy. Radiology 1990;176:345–9.

51. Delongchamps NB, de la Roza G, Jones R, et al. Saturation biopsies on autopsied prostates for detecting and characterizing prostate cancer. BJU Int 2009;103:49–54.

52. Shariat SF, Roehrborn CG. Using biopsy to detect prostate cancer. Rev Urol 2008;10(4):262–80.

53. Heijmink SW, van Moerkerk H, Kiemeney LA, et al. A comparison of the diagnostic performance of systematic versus ultrasound-guided biopsies of prostate cancer. Eur Radiol 2006;16:927–38.

54. Halpern EJ, Ramey JR, Strup SE, et al. Detection of prostate carcinoma with contrast-enhanced sonography using intermittent harmonic imaging. Cancer 2005;104:2373–83.

55. Trabulsi EJ, Sackett D, Gomella LG, et al. Enhanced transrectal ultrasound modalities in the diagnosis of prostate cancer. Urology 2010;76(5): 1025–33.

56. Dominguez-Escrig JL, McCracken SR, Greene D. Beyond diagnosis: evolving prostate biopsy in the era of focal therapy. Prostate Cancer 2011;386207. http://dx.doi.org/10.1155/2011/386207.

57. Eskew LA, Bare RL, McCullough DL. Systematic 5 region prostate biopsy is superior to sextant method for diagnosing carcinoma of the prostate. J Urol 1997;157:199–202.

58. O'Dowd GJ, Miller MC, Orozco R, et al. Analysis of repeated biopsy results within 1 year after a non-cancer diagnosis. Urology 2000;55:553–9.

59. Patel AR, Jones JS, Rabets J, et al. Parasagittal biopsies add minimal information in repeat saturation prostate biopsy. Urology 2004;63:87.

60. Rabets JC, Jones JS, Patel A, et al. Prostate cancer detection with office based saturation biopsy in a repeat biopsy population. J Urol 2004; 172:94.

61. Walz J, Graefen M, Chun FK, et al. High incidence of prostate cancer detected by saturation biopsy after previous negative biopsy series. Eur Urol 2006;50:498.

62. Falzarano SM, Zhou M, Hernandez AV, et al. Can saturation biopsy predict prostate cancer localization in radical prostatectomy specimens: a correlative study and implications for focal therapy. Urology 2010;76:682–7.

63. Ashley RA, Inman BA, Routh JC, et al. Reassessing the diagnostic yield of saturation biopsy of the prostate. Eur Urol 2008;53:976–81.

64. Pepe P, Aragona F. Saturation prostate needle biopsy and prostate cancer detection at initial and repeat evaluation. Urology 2007;70:1131–5.

65. Dimmen M, Vlatkovic L, Hole KH, et al. Transperineal prostate biopsy detects significant cancer in patients with elevated prostate-specific antigen (PSA) levels and previous negative transrectal biopsies. BJU Int 2012;110(2 Pt 2): E69–75.

66. Watanabe M, Hayashi T, Tsushima T, et al. Extensive biopsy using a combined transperineal and transrectal approach to improve prostate cancer detection. Int J Urol 2005;12:959–63.

67. Kawakami S, Okuno T, Yonese J, et al. Optimal sampling sites for repeat prostate biopsy: a recursive partitioning analysis of three-dimensional

26-core systematic biopsy. Eur Urol 2007;51:675–82 [discussion: 682–3].

68. Bott SR, Young MP, Kellett MJ, et al. Anterior prostate cancer: is it more difficult to diagnose? BJU Int 2002;89:886–9.

69. Wright JL, Ellis WJ. Improved prostate cancer detection with anterior apical prostate biopsies. Urol Oncol 2006;24:492–5.

70. Takenaka A, Hara R, Hyodo Y, et al. Transperineal extended biopsy improves the clinically significant prostate cancer detection rate: a comparative study of 6 and 12 biopsy cores. Int J Urol 2006; 13:10–4.

71. Kawakami S, Kihara K, Fujii Y, et al. Transrectal ultrasound-guided transperineal 14-core systematic biopsy detects apico-anterior cancer foci of T1c prostate cancer. Int J Urol 2004;11: 613–8.

72. Shen PF, Zhu YC, Wei WR, et al. The results of transperineal versus transrectal prostate biopsy: a systematic review and meta-analysis. Asian J Androl 2012;14(2):310–5.

73. Pallwein L, Mitterberger M, Pelzer A, et al. Ultrasound of prostate cancer: recent advances. Eur Radiol 2008;18:707–15.

74. Bree RL. The role of color Doppler and staging biopsies in prostate cancer detection. Urology 1997; 49(Suppl 3A):31–4.

75. Mitterberger M, Pinggera G, Horninger W, et al. Comparison of contrast enhanced colour Doppler targeted biopsy to conventional systematic biopsy: impact on Gleason score. J Urol 2007; 178(2):464–8.

76. Mitterberger M, Pinggera G, Horninger W, et al. Dutasteride prior to contrast-enhanced colour Doppler ultrasound prostate biopsy increases prostate cancer detection. Eur Urol 2008;53(1): 112–7.

77. Halpern EJ, Frauscher F, Rosenberg M, et al. Directed biopsy during contrast-enhanced sonography of the prostate. AJR Am J Roentgenol 2002;178(4):915–9.

78. Pelzer A, Bektic J, Berger AP, et al. Prostate cancer detection in men with prostate specific antigen 4 to 10 ng/ml using a combined approach of contrast enhanced color Doppler targeted and systematic biopsy. J Urol 2005;173:1926–9.

79. Krouskop TA, Wheeler TM, Kallel F, et al. Elastic moduli of breast and prostate tissues under compression. Ultrason Imaging 1998;20:260–74.

80. Pallwein L, Mitterberger M, Struve P, et al. Comparison of sonoelastography guided biopsy with systematic biopsy: impact on prostate cancer detection. Eur Radiol 2007;17(9):2278–85.

81. Konig K, Scheipers U, Pesavento A, et al. Initial experiences with real-time elastography guided biopsies of the prostate. J Urol 2005;174:115–7.

82. Pallwein L, Mitterberger M, Pinggera G, et al. Sonoelastography of the prostate: comparison with systematic biopsy findings in 492 patients. Eur J Radiol 2008;65:304–10.

83. Siddiqui MM, Rais-Bahrami S, Truong H, et al. Magnetic resonance imaging/ultrasound-fusion biopsy significantly upgrades prostate cancer versus systematic 12-core transrectal ultrasound biopsy. Eur Urol 2013. http://dx.doi.org/10.1016/j.eururo. 2013.05.059.

84. Pinto PA, Chung PH, Rastinehad AR, et al. Magnetic resonance imaging/ultrasound fusion guided prostate biopsy improves cancer detection following transrectal ultrasound biopsy and correlates with multiparametric magnetic resonance imaging. J Urol 2011;186(4):1281–5.

85. Moore CM, Robertson NL, Arsanious N, et al. Image-guided prostate biopsy using magnetic resonance imaging-derived targets: a systematic review. Eur Urol 2012;63(1):125–40.

86. Marks L, Young S, Natarajan S. MRI-ultrasound fusion for guidance of targeted prostate biopsy. Curr Opin Urol 2013;23(1):43–50.

87. Rodriguez LV, Terris MK. Risks and complications of transrectal ultrasound. Curr Opin Urol 2000;10: 111–6.

88. Toi A. The prostate. In: Rumack CM, Wilson SR, Carboneau WJ, et al, editors. Diagnostic ultrasound. Philadelphia: Elsevier; 2011. p. 392–428.

89. Kapoor DA, Klimberg IW, Malek GH, et al. Single-dose oral ciprofloxacin versus placebo for prophylaxis during transrectal prostate biopsy. Urology 1998;52:552–8.

90. Duplessis CA, Bavaro M, Simons MP, et al. Rectal cultures before transrectal ultrasound-guided prostate biopsy reduce post-prostatic biopsy infection rates. Urology 2012;79(3):556–61.

Prostate Cancer Biomarkers

Marco A. Alvarez, MD

KEYWORDS

- Biomarkers • Prostate • Screening • TRUS • PSA • PCA3 • TMPRSS2:ERG
- Prostate Health Index

KEY POINTS

- Prostate cancer is among the top newly diagnosed cancers in the United States and the rest of the world.
- Its approach has radically shifted because of prostate-specific antigen, transrectal ultrasound-guided biopsy (TRUS), and improvements in medical and surgical options.
- The use of biomarkers for prostate cancer screening helps not only to select which patients will likely benefit from TRUS, thus reducing the need for unnecessary biopsies, but also, once the diagnosis is confirmed, to discriminate between more aggressive and indolent disease, helping to diminish overtreatment.

INTRODUCTION

Prostate cancer (PCa) is among the top newly diagnosed cancers in the United States and the rest of the world.[1,2] Its approach has radically shifted in the past 30 years after the introduction and wide use of prostate-specific antigen (PSA),[3–5] transrectal ultrasound-guided biopsy (TRUS) (**Figs. 1–3**),[6–8] and improvements in the medical and surgical options offered to patients.[9]

To maximize the benefit for the patient, everyone in the team, from the general practitioner, urologist, and radiologist, to the pathologist, must have the basic knowledge and understanding of the tools available and the current trends.[10]

Even despite its current reach and limitations, we believe that the use of biomarkers will revolutionize PCa care. We will move from a one-size-fits-all to a personal tailored approach.

BIOMARKERS

The National Cancer Institute defines a biomarker as "a biological molecule found in blood, other body fluids, or tissues that is a sign of a normal or abnormal process, or a condition, or a disease. A biomarker may be used to see how well the body responds to a treatment for a disease or condition."[11]

An ideal biomarker to screen for PCa, or a combination of them, would improve screening by helping in the decision making as to which patients will likely benefit from a biopsy or rebiopsy. It would also help to differentiate between insignificant and aggressive tumors and guide in the selection of treatment in the case of a positive biopsy and in the long-term management of the disease.[4,10,12–14]

PCa biomarkers can be obtained from urine, blood, and prostate tissue. There is a wide array of options, with no single all-around solution.[15]

PSA

The characteristics of this biomarker (**Fig. 4**) have been widely published and its introduction in the early 1970s resulted in early detection, reducing mortality from PCa.[4,5] Even though its use as a screening tool has been criticized,[16,17] it still has a long future because of many of its characteristics.[18–21]

Diagnostic Radiology and Imaging, Alvarez & Arrazola Radiólogos, Mazatlán, Sinaloa, México
E-mail address: marcoalvarez@gmail.com

Ultrasound Clin 9 (2014) 95–98
http://dx.doi.org/10.1016/j.cult.2013.09.005
1556-858X/14/$ – see front matter © 2014 Elsevier Inc. All rights reserved.

ultrasound.theclinics.com

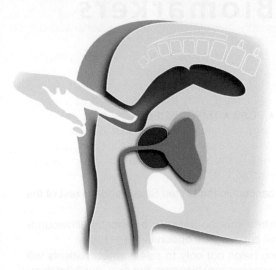

Fig. 1. Digital rectal examination provides information on the state of the peripheral zone of the gland. For centuries, it was the only tool to screen the prostate.

[-2]PROPSA AND PROSTATE HEALTH INDEX

Approved by the US Food and Drug Administration (FDA) in 2012,[22] this PSA isoform, produced in the peripheral zone of the prostate (also known as p2PSA), circulates in the blood as a part of the free PSA fraction and has been used in Europe for several years. It has shown a high accuracy in predicting repeat biopsy outcome,[23] and when used during active surveillance programs, it can also help to predict biopsy reclassification.[24,25] Recent studies have even compared it with other biomarkers, such as PCA3 (Hologic Gen Probe,

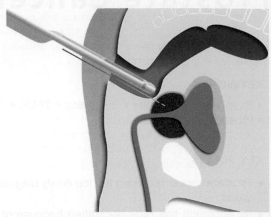

Fig. 3. Prostatic TRUS is the mainstay for diagnosis of PCa.

Bedford, MA, USA), concluding that its use increases both sensitivity and specificity compared with other biomarkers. Its goal is to help reduce the number of unnecessary biopsies.

Through a patented mathematical process, the values of PSA, free PSA, and p2PSA provide the Prostate Health Index (Beckman Coulter, Pasadena CA, USA).[26]

4KSCORE AND PROSTARIX

Other markers, such as 4Kscore (Opko Health, Miami, FL, USA), aim to predict the result of a prostate biopsy. A panel of 4 kallikreins (a subgroup of serine proteases) have been shown to help predict the result of an initial biopsy in previously screened men with increased PSA levels.[27,28]

Prostarix is also a genetic examination, which identifies common PCa alleles and aims to provide population risk stratification.[29]

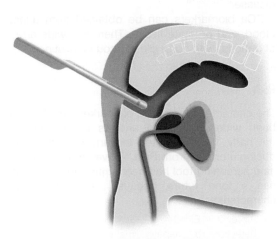

Fig. 2. TRUS was introduced in the 1980s and provides real-time anatomic views of the prostate. Recent advances in sonography, such as the use of contrast and elastography, are being tested to improve its efficacy.

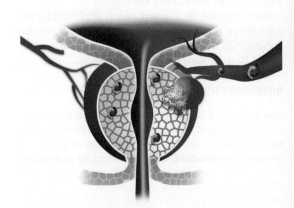

Fig. 4. PSA was introduced in the early 1970s and has been at the forefront for PCa screening. The use of some of its derivatives, such as [-2]proPSA, has improved its value.

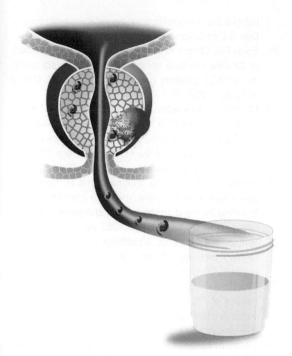

Fig. 5. Biomarkers, such as PCA3, will revolutionize PCa care. We will move from a one-size-fits-all to a personal tailored approach.

PCA3

Available in urine, the PCA3 is a biomarker used to screen for PCa (**Fig. 5**). Its a noncoding prostate-specific messenger RNA, which can be found in urine and prostatic fluid and is overexpressed only in PCa[30–35] Benign prostate hypertrophy and inflammatory conditions do not affect the PCA3 values.[36]

Even though it is FDA approved to guide the decision whether to perform a repeat biopsy, in Europe, it has been used to inform the initial biopsy decision with better results than PSA.[37,38] It has been found to be more discriminatory than PSA and can reduce the number of unnecessary prostate biopsies, but further evidence is needed to prove that it can improve health outcomes.[31,33] Its efficiency in detecting high-grade intraepithelial neoplasia is lower than in men with benign hypertrophy,[39] but its value is not influenced by chronic prostatitis.[40]

TMPRSS2:ERG

This common chromosomal aberration has a high specificity for PCa diagnosis and can be found in samples from urine and tissue.[41] It has been used in conjunction with PCA3 to try to predict PCa at time of biopsy.[42]

Several other biomarkers, such as ConfirmMDx, Prolaris, Oncotype Dx, Metamark, ProstaVysion,

Decipher, and ProsVue, are also being researched, making this topic a work in progress.

SUMMARY

It remains to be seen which of these biomarkers, or a combination of them, will most affect clinical decision making, because there is a legitimate need to validate data. We should not aim to perform more TRUS biopsies but to select better those patients who are candidates for one.

The use of biomarkers as well as state-of-the-art imaging techniques promise to improve screening not only to detect PCa but also to identify those patients who will likely benefit from treatment. This development will provide an opportunity to revolutionize the care of patients with PCa. With continuing progress, it will be possible to offer patients a tailored approach (a smarter screening and selective treatment).

REFERENCES

1. Brawley OW. Prostate cancer epidemiology in the United States. World J Urol 2012;30(2):195–200.
2. Available at: http://www.cancer.org/acs/groups/content/@epidemiologysurveilance/documents/document/acspc-036845.pdf.
3. Partin AW. Early detection of prostate cancer continues to support rational, limited screening. J Urol 2013;190:427–8.
4. Bjartell A. Next generation prostate-specific antigen test: ready to use? Eur Urol 2013. [Epub ahead of print].
5. Marberger M. Current prostate cancer: 20 years later. BJU Int 2007;100(Suppl 2):11–4.
6. Martínez-Ballesteros C, Mtz Salamanca J, Carbadillo J. Prostatic biopsy: responsibility diagnosed and recent changes. Arch Esp Urol 2011;64(8):735–45.
7. Kelloff G, Choyke P, Coffey D. Challenges in clinical prostate cancer: role of imaging. AJR Am J Roentgenol 2009;192:1455–70.
8. Stoianovici D. Technology advances for prostate biopsy and needle therapies. J Urol 2012;188:1074–5.
9. Madan R, Arlen P. Recent advances revolutionize treatment of metastatic prostate cancer. Future Oncol 2013;9(8):1133–44.
10. Ballentine C, Albertsen P, Barry M, et al. Early detection of prostate cancer: AUA Guideline. J Urol 2013;190:419–26.
11. Available at: http://www.cancer.gov/dictionary?cdrid=45618.
12. Laskiewicz L, Altieri D, Jiang Z, et al. The search for a better prostate cancer biomarker. J Urol 2011;186:1758–9.

13. Schiffer E. Biomarkers for prostate cancer. World J Urol 2007;25:557–62.

14. Steuber T, Helo P, Lilja H. Circulating biomarkers for prostate cancer. World J Urol 2007;25(2):111–9.

15. Prior C, Robles J, Catena R, et al. Use of a combination of biomarkers in serum and urine to improve detection of prostate cancer. World J Urol 2010;6: 681–6.

16. Chou R, Croswell JM, Dana T, et al. Screening for prostate cancer: a review of the evidence for the US Preventive Services Task Force. Ann Intern Med 2011;1555:762–71.

17. Available at: http://www.nytimes.com/2010/03/10/opinion/10Ablin.html.

18. Vickers A, Scardino P, Hugosson J, et al. Prostate cancer screening: facts, statistics, and interpretation in response to the US preventive service task force review. J Clin Oncol 2012;30(21):2581–4.

19. Catalona W, Loeb S. The PSA era is not over for prostate cancer. Eur Urol 2005;48:541–5.

20. Clements R. Prostate specific antigen: an opinion on its value to the radiologist. Eur Radiol 1998;9: 529–35.

21. Thompson I, Tangen C. Prostate cancer–uncertainty and way forward. N Engl J Med 2012;367(3):270–1.

22. Available at: http://www.fda.gov/MedicalDevices/ProductsandMedicalProcedures/DeviceApprovalsandClearances/Recently-ApprovedDevices/ucm309081.html.

23. Lazzeri M, Briganti A, Scattoni V, et al. Serum Index Test %[-2]proPSA and prostate health index are more accurate than prostate specific antigen and %fPSA in predicting a positive repeat prostate biopsy. J Urol 2012;188:1137–43.

24. Tosoian J, Loeb S, Feng Z, et al. Association of [-2] proPSA with biopsy reclassification during active surveillance for prostate cancer. J Urol 2012;188: 1131–6.

25. Scattoni V, Lazzeri M, Lughezzani G, et al. Head to head comparison of prostate health index and urinary PCA3 for predicting cancer at initial or repeat biopsy. J Urol 2013;190:496–501.

26. Hansen F, van Schaik R, Kurstjens J, et al. Prostate-specific antigen (PSA) isoform p2PSA in combination with total PSA and free PSA improves diagnostic accuracy in prostate cancer detection. Eur Urol 2010;57:e53–68.

27. Vickers AJ, Cronin AM, Roobol MJ, et al. A four-kallikrein panel predicts prostate cancer in men with recent screening: data from the European Randomized. Study of screening for prostate cancer, Rotterdam. Clin Cancer Res 2010;16(12): 3232–9.

28. Vickers A, Cronin A, Roobol M, et al. Reducing unnecessary biopsy during prostate cancer screening using a four-kallikrein panel: an independent replication. J Clin Oncol 2010;28(15):2493–8.

29. Eeles RA, Olama AA, Benlloch S, et al. Identification of 23 new prostate cancer susceptibility loci using the iCOGS custom genotyping array. Nat Genet 2013;45(4):385–91.

30. Martínez J, Saavedra- Briones D, Rodriguez M, et al. Development of PCA3 urinary test inexpensive and initial experience for the detection of prostate cancer in Mexican patients at the Hospital General Dr. Manuel Gea Gonzalez. Rev Mex Urol 2010;70(5):328–35.

31. Bradley L, Palomaki G, Gutman S, et al. Comparative effectiveness review: prostate cancer antigen 3 testing for the diagnosis and management of prostate cancer. J Urol 2013;190:389–98.

32. Ruffon A, André J, Vlaeminck-Guillem V, et al. Urinary prostate cancer 3 test: toward the age of reason? Urology 2010;75:447–53.

33. Crawford D, Rove K, Qian J, et al. Diagnostic performance of PCA3 to detect prostate cancer in men with increased prostate specific antigen: a prospective study of 1,962 cases. J Urol 2012;188:1726–31.

34. Deras E, Blase A, Day R, et al. PCA3: a molecular urine assay for predicting prostate biopsy outcome. J Urol 2008;179:1587–92.

35. Ruiz- Aragón J, Marquez- Pelaes S. Evaluation of the PCA3 test for the diagnosis of prostate cancer: systematic review and meta-analysis. Actas Urol Esp 2010;34:346–55 [in Spanish].

36. Vlaeminck-Guillen V, Bandel M, Cottancin M. Re: Chronic prostatitis does not influence urinary PCA3 score. J Urol 2012;188:2242–5.

37. De la Taille A, Irani J, Chun F, et al. Clinical evaluation of the PCA3 assay in guiding initial biopsy decisions. J Urol 2011;185:2119–25.

38. Tombal B, Ameye F, Gontero P, et al. Biopsy and treatment decisions in the initial management of prostate cancer and role of PCA3; a systematic analysis of expert opinion. World J Urol 2011;30(2): 251–6.

39. Morote J, Rigau M, Ballesteros C, et al. Behavior of the PCA3 gene in the urine of men with high grade prostatic intraepithelial neoplasia. World J Urol 2010;28(6):677–80.

40. Vlaeminck- Guillen V, Bandel M, Cottancin M, et al. Infection and inflammation of the genitourinary tract. Re: chronic prostatitis does not influence urinary PCA3 score. J Urol 2012;188:2242–5.

41. Perner S, Mosquera JM, Paris P, et al. TMPRSS2-ERG fusion prostate cancer: an early molecular event associated with invasion. Am J Surg Pathol 2007;31:882–8.

42. Salagierski M, Schalken J. Molecular diagnosis of prostate cancer: PCA3 and TMPRSS2: ERG gene fusion. J Urol 2011;187:795–801.

Salivary Gland: Oncologic Imaging

Uday Y. Mandalia, MBBS, BSc, MRCPCH, FRCR[a],*,
Francois N. Porte, MBBS, FRCR[a],
David C. Howlett, FRCP, FRCR[b]

KEYWORDS

- Salivary gland • Neoplasm • Ultrasound • Ultrasound-guided biopsy

KEY POINTS

- Salivary gland neoplasms constitute a wide range of benign and malignant disorders and imaging constitutes an integral part of the initial assessment of a suspected salivary gland lesion.
- Because of their location, the salivary glands are readily accessible with high-resolution ultrasound, which is considered the first-line imaging modality in many centers.
- By providing information regarding the site, nature, and extent of disorder, ultrasound can characterize a lesion with a high degree of sensitivity and specificity.
- Ultrasound can also be used for image-guided interventions with fine-needle aspiration cytology or core biopsy.
- Ultrasound provides a guide if further imaging with computed tomography or magnetic resonance imaging are required.

ANATOMY OF THE PAROTID SPACE

The parotid gland lies in the retromandibular fossa and is bordered posteriorly by the sternocleidomastoid muscle and posteromedially by the mastoid process. The masseter and medial pterygoid muscles are located anteromedial to the gland, along with the mandibular ramus. The gland consists of superficial and deep lobes, which are defined by the path of the facial nerve traveling through the gland. The superficial lobe is readily imaged with high-frequency ultrasound, although the deep lobe cannot be easily visualized in its entirety, because it is partially obscured by the mandible.[1] The facial nerve is also not usually identified on ultrasound; however, its position can be inferred because it passes in a plane just superficial to the adjacent retromandibular vein (RMV). Hence, identification of the RMV allows compartmentalization into superficial and deep lobes. Lying inferior to the retromandibular vein is the external carotid artery, which branches into the maxillary and superficial temporal arteries within the gland (**Figs. 1** and **2**).

The parotid duct, or Stensen duct, exits the gland anteriorly, passes above the masseter muscle, and perforates the buccal fat and buccinator muscle to open into the oral cavity at the level of the second upper molar. Accessory parotid tissue may be found along the course of the parotid duct, arising in approximately 20% of the population.[2] The parotid gland is predominantly a serous gland.

The parotid gland becomes encapsulated later embryologically than the submandibular and sublingual glands, and therefore intraglandular lymph nodes may be found within it. These nodes tend to be located in the preauricular portion of the gland or within the parotid tail. A normal parotid lymph node is oval or kidney shaped with a smooth contour; has a central, echo-bright fatty hilum; and contains a feeding hilar vessel that can be seen on color Doppler ultrasound.

[a] Guys and St Thomas' NHS Trust, Radiology Department, St Thomas' Hospital, Westminster Bridge Road, London SE1 7EH, UK; [b] Brighton and Sussex Medical School, Kings College London, East Sussex Hospitals NHS Trust, Radiology Department, Eastbourne District General Hospital, Kings Drive, Eastbourne, East Sussex BN21 2UD, UK
* Corresponding author.
E-mail address: udaymandalia@hotmail.com

Ultrasound Clin 9 (2014) 99–113
http://dx.doi.org/10.1016/j.cult.2013.08.005
1556-858X/14/$ – see front matter © 2014 Elsevier Inc. All rights reserved.

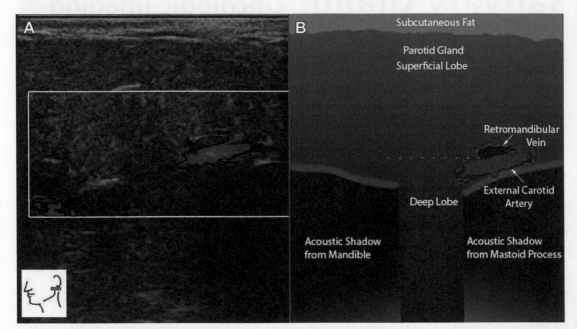

Fig. 1. Transverse sonogram of the left parotid (*A*) with corresponding schematic diagram (*B*), showing the position of the retromandibular vein, allowing compartmentalization into superficial and deep lobes. The probe position is seen in the inset diagram.

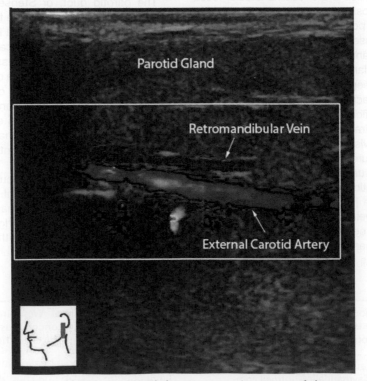

Fig. 2. Longitudinal sonogram of the left parotid showing normal anatomy of the retromandibular vein and external carotid artery.

ANATOMY OF THE SUBMANDIBULAR GLAND

The submandibular gland lies in the space located inferior to the body of the mandible and between the anterior and posterior bellies of the digastric muscle. The gland is roughly triangular in shape and, like the parotid gland, is made up of superficial and deep lobes, although these are of less clinical significance than the parotid gland. The submandibular gland does not contain lymph nodes, although lymph nodes are found within the submandibular space superior and anterior to the gland.[3]

The facial artery arises from the external carotid artery and passes through a groove on the posteroinferior aspect the submandibular gland. The facial artery may pass through the parenchyma of the gland.[3] The facial vein crosses over the superficial aspect of the gland. The marginal mandibular nerve also crosses the gland superficially, within the deep cervical fascia. The submandibular duct (or Wharton duct) originates from multiple ductal branches situated on the deep aspect of the gland, extends anteriorly between the mylohyoid and hypoglossus muscles, crosses the medial aspect of the sublingual gland, and drains into the mouth at the sublingual caruncle, situated on the frenulum lingulae. The submandibular gland is a mixed serous/mucinous gland.

ANATOMY OF THE SUBLINGUAL GLAND

The sublingual gland is the smallest of the 3 major salivary glands. It is situated posterior to the mandible and lies below the mucous membrane of the floor of the mouth. The gland is bordered inferiorly by the mylohyoid muscle and medially by the genioglossus and the submandibular duct. The sublingual gland has a variable number of excretory ducts, many of which drain directly into the floor of the mouth, although some ducts form the sublingual duct of Bartholin, which joins the submandibular duct to drain into the sublingual caruncle. The gland can be visualized on ultrasound when scanning in the submental region and appears as an echogenic oval-shaped structure on transverse imaging.[3] The sublingual gland is a predominantly mucinous gland.

CLINICAL PRESENTATION OF A SALIVARY GLAND TUMOR

Major salivary gland tumors present as painless masses in the region of the affected salivary gland. Benign tumors are usually slow growing, whereas malignant tumors vary in their rate of growth depending on their grade, although a sudden painful increase in size may also be related to infarction (Fig. 3). Pain is a poor discriminator between benign

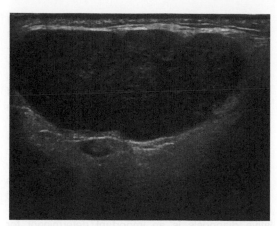

Fig. 3. Sonogram of the right parotid mass in the superficial lobe. This mass is hypoechoic and inhomogeneous. The lesion was painful and had enlarged rapidly, and biopsy confirmed an infarcted Warthin tumor.

and malignant disease because it is experienced in 5.1% of patients with benign tumors and 6.5% of patients with malignant disease.[4,5] However, in patients with proven salivary gland carcinoma, the presence of pain is a poor prognostic indicator, because it signifies perineural spread of disease, which is associated with a 5-year reduction in survival from 68% to 35%. Cranial nerve VII is most commonly involved because of its course through the parotid, thus symptoms include facial pain and facial nerve paralysis. With progressive tumor invasion other cranial nerves may become involved.[6,7]

Lymph node metastases from a salivary gland tumor may present as a firm enlarging neck lump. The primary drainage for the parotid and submandibular glands is to the deep cervical chain, whereas the sublingual gland drains to submental and submandibular nodes. Nodal metastases are associated with a poorer prognosis, with an associated reduction in 10-year survival from 63% to 33%.[8]

Distant metastasis is also an indicator of poor prognosis and is seen in 20% of the parotid cancers, most commonly from adenoid cystic carcinoma, followed by undifferentiated carcinoma.[6]

THE ROLE OF IMAGING

The diagnosis of a salivary gland tumor ideally is based on the concept of triple assessment:

1. Clinical evaluation
2. Imaging
3. Histologic/cytologic evaluation

Although salivary gland tumors are rare and usually benign, surgical excision represents the treatment of choice in most circumstances. Imaging is needed not only to confirm the presence of a lesion but also to determine its spread, intraglandular/extraglandular extent, identification of clinically occult lesions, as well as unsuspected cervical lymphadenopathy. The imaging characteristics of a lesion can determine whether a tumor is benign or malignant with a high sensitivity and specificity.[9] An accurate preoperative diagnosis of a parotid lesion is critical because many nonneoplastic lesions do not require surgery. The need for surgery may also be avoided in certain benign neoplasms (eg, Warthin tumors) or if the patient is considered too elderly or unfit for surgery. An accurate preoperative diagnosis is an important determinant for operative planning, notably with the increased use of extracapsular, parotid-sparing dissection and to allow appropriate informed patient consent (in particular pertaining to facial nerve integrity and also possible nodal dissection in malignancy).[10,11]

Ultrasound is frequently accepted as the initial imaging modality of choice.[12] It has the advantages of being portable and allowing multiplanar, noninvasive imaging without the need of ionizing radiation. High-frequency linear array probes are capable of producing high-resolution images of the salivary glands with a spatial resolution surpassing computed tomography (CT) and magnetic resonance (MR) imaging. However, compared with these modalities, ultrasound has some disadvantages: it is operator dependent and is limited in visualization of large lesions or those extending into the deep lobe of the parotid because of obscuration by the mandible.[13]

Most lesions lie within the superficial lobe and ultrasound is usually able to compartmentalize a lesion according to its relationship to intraparotid vessels and the inferred position of the facial nerve. For large or suspected malignant lesions and lesions of the deep lobe of the parotid gland, MR imaging or CT are the modalities of choice; however, even in these cases, ultrasound can act as an indicator for additional investigation.[13,14]

Following the initial sonographic diagnosis of a salivary gland tumor, ultrasound-guided biopsy (with fine-needle aspiration cytology [FNAC] or ultrasound-guided core biopsy [USCB]; discussed later) is a safe and reliable method of obtaining the histopathologic confirmation of a lesion necessary to instruct further surgical management.[15–17] The goals of imaging salivary gland tumors can be seen in **Box 1**.

SONOGRAPHIC TECHNIQUE

A high-frequency linear array transducer, typically 7 to 12 MHz or greater, should be used in the

---

Box 1
The aims of imaging in salivary gland tumors

1. Localization of the lesion
2. Determination of the nature of the lesion
3. Tumor staging for preoperative planning
4. Detection of cervical lymphadenopathy
5. Image-guided biopsy

---

assessment of the salivary glands. A lower frequency transducer (5–10 MHz) can be used to assess large tumors fully and to visualize lesions located in the deeper aspects of the glands.[18–20]

To facilitate visualization, a pillow or towel can placed under the patient's shoulders to extend the patient's neck. The salivary glands and any lesion discovered within them should be interrogated in at least 2 perpendicular planes. An oblique approach may be required to navigate around the mandible. The contralateral salivary gland needs to be examined for comparison and to look for bilateral disease. To complete the study, the entire neck should be imaged for related disorders and lymph node enlargement. Color Doppler assessment provides information regarding the vascular resistance and flow pattern of a lesion, which can improve diagnostic accuracy for malignant tumors.[21]

SALIVARY GLAND NEOPLASTIC DISEASE

When all salivary gland tumors are considered, the global incidence varies from 0.4 to 13.5 cases per 100,000 population.[22] About 80% of all lesions are benign, hence salivary malignancies are rare entities, comprising less than 0.5% of all malignancies and about 5% of cancers of the head and neck.[23] They constitute a wide variety of disorders (**Table 1**). They are divided into benign and malignant neoplasms, which can be epithelial or nonepithelial in origin. The parotid gland contains 70% of all salivary gland tumors, with 8% found in the submandibular glands and 22% in the minor glands.[24]

There are some general rules that apply to salivary gland neoplasms. The smaller the salivary gland, the higher the rate of malignancy. Thus, the rate of malignancy increases from 20% to 25% in the parotid gland to 40% to 50% in the submandibular gland, and to 50% to 81% in the sublingual glands and minor salivary glands.[25–28]

Environmental and genetic factors have been proposed as causes of salivary gland neoplasms. The strongest link seems to be with radiation exposure and smoking, which have been implicated in the development of Warthin tumors.[29]

Table 1
World Health Organization classification of epithelial salivary gland neoplasms

Benign Epithelial Tumors	Malignant Epithelial Tumors
Pleomorphic adenoma	Acinic cell carcinoma
Myoepithelioma	Mucoepidermoid carcinoma
Basal cell adenoma	Adenoid cystic carcinoma
Warthin tumor	Polymorphous low-grade adenocarcinoma
Oncocytoma	Epithelial-myoepithelial carcinoma
Canalicular adenoma	Clear cell carcinoma, not otherwise specified
Sebaceous adenoma	Basal cell adenocarcinoma
Lymphadenoma	Sebaceous carcinoma
Sebaceous nonsebaceous ductal papilloma	Sebaceous lymphadenocarcinoma
Inverted ductal papilloma	Cystadenocarcinoma
Intraductal papilloma	Low-grade cribriform cystadenocarcinoma
Sialadenoma papilliferum	Mucinous adenocarcinoma
Cystadenoma	Oncocytic carcinoma
	Salivary duct carcinoma
	Adenocarcinoma not otherwise specified
	Myoepithelial carcinoma
	Carcinoma ex pleomorphic adenoma
	Carcinosarcoma
	Metastasizing pleomorphic adenoma
	Squamous cell carcinoma
	Small cell carcinoma
	Large cell carcinoma
	Lymphoepithelial carcinoma
	Sialoblastoma
	Soft tissue tumors
	Hemangioma
	Hematolymphoid tumors
	Hodgkin lymphoma
	Diffuse large B-cell lymphoma
	Extranodal marginal zone B-cell lymphoma
	Secondary tumors

Data from Barnes L, Eveson JW, Reichart P, Sidransky D, editors. World Health Organization classification of tumours: pathology and genetics, head and neck tumours. Lyon: IARC Press; 2005. p. 242–3.

BENIGN TUMORS

About 65% of all salivary gland tumors are pleomorphic adenomas, followed by Warthin tumor in 3.5% to 30% depending on geographic location. The remainder are rare benign tumors.[30] On ultrasound these lesions typically appear as smooth, round, hypoechoic masses with distal acoustic enhancement (**Fig. 4**). These tumors may appear lobulated. Large tumors may appear more heterogeneous than small ones and may require further evaluation with MR imaging.

PLEOMORPHIC ADENOMAS

Pleomorphic adenomas represent the most common benign parotid and submandibular tumor. They are of mixed cell origin with considerable variation in the myoepithelial, mesenchymal, and epithelial components. They usually present as slow-growing, asymptomatic masses in middle-aged patients. Pleomorphic adenomas occur most often in people in the fourth and fifth decades of life but may arise at any age. They have a slight female preponderance. About 80% of pleomorphic adenomas arise in the parotid; 10% in the submandibular gland; and 10% in the minor salivary glands of the oral cavity, nasal cavity, and paranasal sinuses and the upper respiratory and alimentary tracts.[24] Of the parotid lesions, 90% occur in the superficial lobe, frequently in the tail. They are usually solitary and unilateral.[22,31]

If left untreated, approximately 5% undergo malignant transformation, usually after a period of decades.[4,22] In view of their malignant potential, surgical resection is the mainstay of treatment. Pleomorphic adenomas treated by surgical enucleation or those that experience intraoperative rupture or transection have a high rate of multifocal local recurrence, and they can rarely behave aggressively, showing metastatic spread.[32]

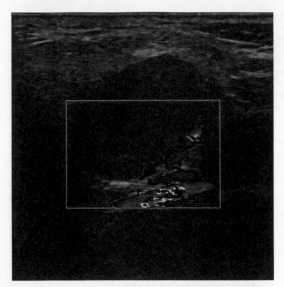

Fig. 4. Sonogram of a parotid pleomorphic adenoma. The lesion is hypoechoic, reasonably homogeneous, and well circumscribed. There is distal acoustic enhancement. Note the relationship to the intraparotid vessels deep to the lesion, locating the lesion to the superficial lobe.

On ultrasound, pleomorphic adenomas are characteristically hypoechoic, well-defined, lobulated tumors with posterior acoustic enhancement (see **Fig. 4**). Larger tumors may appear poorly defined with cystic degeneration and internal heterogeneity and can be mistaken for malignancy (**Fig. 5**). Multifocal primary lesions have also been reported.[33] The homogeneity of internal echoes has been regarded as a typical feature of pleomorphic adenoma; however, it is likely to depend on tumor composition.[34–36] Dystrophic calcifications may also form in long-standing lesions and are best visualized with CT.[37–39]

WARTHIN TUMOR (CYSTADENOLYMPHOMA)

Warthin tumor is the second most common benign neoplasm of the salivary gland. It is exclusively found in the parotid and accounts for 20% of all epithelial parotid tumors. It arises from heterotopic parotid tissue within parotid lymph nodes. These tumors present as slow-growing masses within the superficial lobe of the parotid near the angle of the mandible. They are most commonly found in elderly men in the fifth to sixth decade and are associated with smoking and ionizing radiation. Warthin tumors can be bilateral or multiple in 15% of patients. Tumors are metachronous in 75% of multifocal cases.[22,31,40]

On sonography, these tumors are rounded or lobulated hypoechoic masses that may show cystic

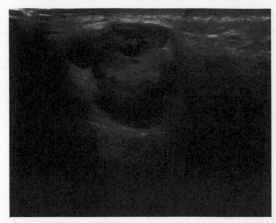

Fig. 5. Sonogram of the right parotid shows a large hypoechoic mass, inhomogeneous and ill defined in parts. This lesion had some sonographically suspicious features, but biopsy confirmed pleomorphic adenoma. As these lesions enlarge they can appear atypical/malignant on ultrasound with ill-defined margins and internal calcification, and cystic change may also be apparent.

change with hyperechoic internal septation. They may present as entirely cystic structures, requiring differentiation from other benign and malignant cystic lesions (**Figs. 6–8**).[3,4,41] Biopsy of these tumors can be challenging because of the paucity of solid material; however, core biopsies through the tumor wall may allow histologic diagnosis.

On MR imaging these tumors are homogenous to intermediate signal on T1. On T2-weighted imaging they are intermediate signal with focal hyperintense areas corresponding with cystic components. A characteristic feature of Warthin tumors is their lack of enhancement with gadolinium.[42,43] Warthin tumors show increased tracer uptake on 99mTc scintigraphy.[44]

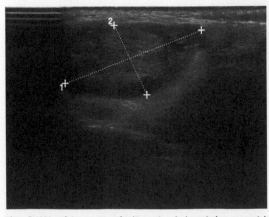

Fig. 6. Warthin tumor (calipers) of the right parotid. Note the inhomogeneous internal architecture and cystic changes.

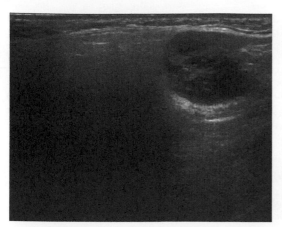

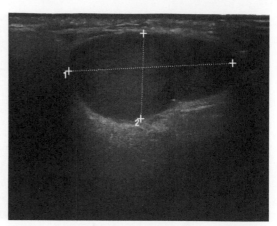

Fig. 7. Sonogram of the left parotid (same patient as in **Fig. 6**) shows a contralateral Warthin tumor.

Fig. 9. Sonogram of an oncocytoma; sonographic features are similar to those associated with a pleomorphic adenoma.

ONCOCYTOMA

Oncocytoma is an uncommon, benign salivary neoplasm composed of mitochondria-rich epithelial cells called oncocytes. They account for about 1% of all the salivary gland neoplasms.[26] Most (84%) cases occur in the parotid gland,[45] with the remainder occurring in the submandibular and minor glands. They present as slow-growing, painless, mobile masses usually within the superficial lobe of the gland.[41]

Oncocytoma has similar imaging characteristics to pleomorphic adenoma. On ultrasound these lesions appear well circumscribed and lobulated (**Fig. 9**).[4,41]

OTHER BENIGN NONEPITHELIAL TUMORS

Hemangiomas of the salivary glands account for approximately 0.4% of salivary tumors.[46] Lesions

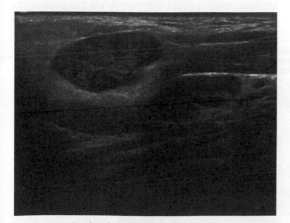

Fig. 8. Longitudinal sonogram of a Warthin tumor in the lower pole of the parotid gland. The lesion is hypoechoic and inhomogeneous but well circumscribed and there is distal acoustic enhancement. The sonographic appearances are similar to those associated with pleomorphic adenoma.

may present at any age but two-thirds of cases are diagnosed in the first 2 decades. They are the most common type of pediatric salivary gland tumor arising in infancy and undergo involution usually by the age of 9 years. They are twice as common in female patients as in male patients.[46,47] Hemangiomas of the parotid appear solid and hypoechoic on ultrasound. On color Doppler imaging they show prominent internal vascularity. Calcified phleboliths are commonly seen within these tumors.[21]

Lipomas of the salivary glands are rare; however, they can occur in the parotid and account for approximately 1% to 2% of all parotid neoplasms.[48] On sonography the lesions are usually well defined but can also appear ill defined. They are normally hypoechoic and contain internal echogenic foci or striations.[49]

MALIGNANT LESION

Sonographic features that suggest a malignant lesion are ill-defined borders, hypoechoic and heterogeneous architecture with distal acoustic shadowing, and extraglandular extension (**Figs. 10–12**).

MUCOEPIDERMOID CARCINOMA

Mucoepidermoid carcinoma is the most common primary malignancy of the salivary glands, representing 20% of all salivary gland malignancies. They arise from ductal epithelium.[22,25] Approximately half of tumors (53%) occur in major glands, most frequently in the parotid gland, representing 45%, with 7% in the submandibular glands, and 1% in sublingual glands. The most frequent intraoral sites are the palate and buccal mucosa.[30] Lesions tend to occur in middle-aged adults (35–65 years). Sonographic features depend on the histologic grade of the tumor. Most tumors

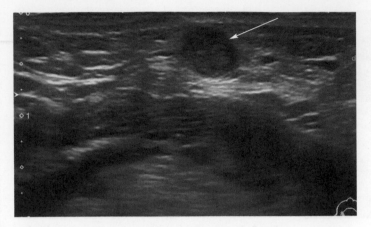

Fig. 10. Sonogram in a patient with a hard nodule in the right submandibular region. The patient had a previous history of a low-grade adenocarcinoma of the right submandibular gland. Ultrasound shows an ill-defined, heterogeneous, hypoechoic solid nodule (*arrow*) that was confirmed as recurrent tumor on biopsy.

are low to intermediate grade, and have a good prognosis with surgery. However, high-grade tumors have a poorer prognosis and increased metastatic potential.[22]

Lower grade lesions appear well defined and may display a lobulated shape with homogenous internal architecture, displaying significant overlap with pleomorphic adenomas both sonographically and clinically (**Fig. 13**). High-grade aggressive lesions are poorly defined, with an irregular shape; blurred margin; and hypoechoic, heterogeneous internal architecture (**Fig. 14**). Tumors may be predominantly cystic or mixed cystic with solid mural components.[9,36,50] Once biopsy has confirmed diagnosis, MR imaging is necessary to complete locoregional staging and a CT of the chest to look for metastatic spread.

ADENOID CYSTIC CARCINOMA

Adenoid cystic carcinoma is the second most common parotid malignancy. It accounts for 2%

to 6% of parotid gland tumors and is the most common submandibular and minor salivary gland malignancy.[25]

The tumor presents as a painful slow-growing mass. The tumor is unencapsulated and may appear well circumscribed on ultrasound. These tumors have a tendency for perineural and local invasion, which explains the high incidence of associated facial pain (33%) and facial nerve paralysis. Late recurrence can occur up to 20 years after treatment. Perineural invasion can be accurately assessed with multiplanar MR imaging and abnormal neural enhancement and skull base extension may be seen after contrast.[47,51]

METASTASIS

The parotid gland contains lymphatic tissues and lymph nodes because of its late encapsulation, within which metastatic disease may occur. Metastatic spread is most commonly via the scalp lymphatics with squamous carcinoma (37%) and

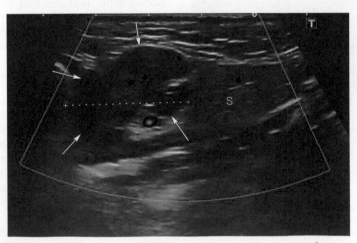

Fig. 11. Sonogram of the right submandibular gland (S) shows an ill-defined mass of mixed echotexture (*arrows*) arising from the lateral aspect of the gland. Biopsy confirmed malignancy.

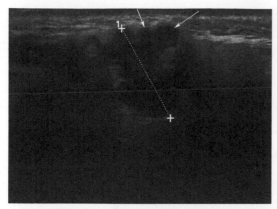

Fig. 12. Sonogram of an acinic cell carcinoma of the right parotid gland (calipers). The lesion is ill defined, heterogeneous, and hypoechoic. Note the extracapsular extension (*arrows*).

melanoma (46%) being the most common primaries.[52] Less commonly lung, renal, or breast carcinoma can spread hematogenously to the parotid gland.[53,54] On ultrasound, metastases vary in appearance: lesions tend to be hypoechoic, with heterogeneous internal architecture and ill-defined margins (**Fig. 15**).[55]

LYMPHOMA

Primary salivary gland lymphoma is rare, accounting for only 5% of all primary extranodal lymphomas and 2% of all salivary gland tumors.[56]

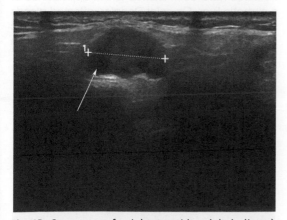

Fig. 13. Sonogram of a right parotid nodule (calipers). The lesion lies in the superficial lobe, it is circumscribed and hypoechoic. There is distal acoustic enhancement and the internal architecture is mildly inhomogeneous, with a poorly hypoechoic focus present (*arrow*). On ultrasound, the lesion appears likely to be benign, with features consistent with a pleomorphic adenoma. However, biopsy confirmed a low-grade mucoepidermoid carcinoma. Small, low-grade malignancies can mimic benign tumors both clinically and sonographically.

The most commonly affected gland is the parotid gland (75%), followed by the submandibular gland (20%). Most lymphomas occurring in salivary glands are mucosa-associated lymphoid tissue (MALT) lymphomas, which are low-grade B-cell non-Hodgkin lymphomas (NHL) that often develop in the setting of chronic lymphoepithelial sialadenitis seen in patients with Sjögren syndrome (**Figs. 16** and **17**).[57,58] Primary and secondary non-MALT lymphomas of the salivary glands may also occur and involvement can be in the form of focal nodal disease or diffuse infiltration of the gland.[39,59]

The imaging features of parotid lymphoma are variable. Focal lymphomatous nodes may have a pseudocystic or micronodular pattern (**Fig. 18**), whereas diffuse involvement may present as generalized enlargement of the gland. There may be associated regional lymphadenopathy and glandular sialectasis. Diffuse disease may manifest with a pattern of multiple hypoechoic lesions with increased vascularity. In these circumstances, differentiation from benign inflammatory conditions is required.[60,61]

CARCINOMA EX PLEOMORPHIC ADENOMAS

There are 3 types of malignancies that occur within preexisting pleomorphic adenomas. The most common is the carcinoma ex pleomorphic adenoma, which originates from epithelial cells; these represent 12% of all malignant salivary gland tumors. The other two forms are true malignant mixed tumor (carcinosarcoma) and metastasizing pleomorphic adenoma.[62,63] Concerning features of malignant degeneration are pain and a sudden increase in size within a long-standing mass. However, this is also seen in tumor infarction (see **Fig. 3**). The rate of occurrence increases with the period the pleomorphic adenoma is left untreated. According to some investigators, the rate of malignant change is 1.5% in the first year in which the adenoma goes untreated, and increases to 9.5% after 15 years.[64,65]

On imaging they look similar to a pleomorphic adenoma, or may show infiltrative margins, necrotic areas, and regional lymph node involvement.

COLOR FLOW ASSESSMENT

Malignant lesions tend to show increased, disordered, and chaotic vascularity compared with benign lesion. Various studies have used different markers of vascularity to differentiate between benign and malignant salivary gland tumors. Some studies have shown that highly vascular lesions and those with a high systolic peak flow velocity (>25 cm/s) are suspicious of malignancy,

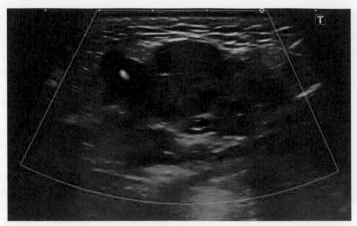

Fig. 14. Mucoepidermoid carcinoma of the left submandibular gland. A large hypoechoic solid mass with ill-defined margins, relatively avascular, replaces normal gland architecture.

regardless of the gray-scale appearance of the tumor. However, measurement of peak systolic velocity in small intratumoral vessels is imprecise, and doubts have been raised regarding the ability to accurately angle correct on small intratumoral vessels.[66,67]

Other studies have measured the vascular resistance of intratumoral vessels, showing that tumors with an increased resistance have an increased risk of malignancy. In those with high pulsatility index (PI) and resistive index (RI), the risk of malignancy increases by a third (PI>1.8 and RI>0.8).[21]

TUMOR MIMICS

Pseudotumors are mimics of salivary gland tumors. Lymphadenopathy in the region of the salivary glands can be misinterpreted as a mass of salivary gland origin. This mass may be secondary to inflammatory conditions such as sarcoid or nodal metastases from head and neck cancers (**Fig. 19**).

Another important example is the Kuttner tumor, a form of chronic sclerosing sialadenitis, presenting as a firm, painful swelling of 1 or both submandibular glands. The disorder is characterized by plasmocytic and lymphocytic periductal infiltrates, which eventually lead to encasement of ducts with fibrotic tissue.[68] On ultrasound, the gland appears diffusely hypoechoic and heterogeneous with multiple small hypoechoic foci with background heterogeneity. Features have been likened to the appearance of a cirrhotic liver. On color Doppler, affected glands showed prominent vascularity.[69] The sonographic appearances are typical and biopsy confirmation is often not required (**Fig. 20**).

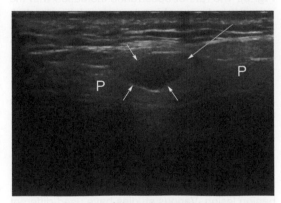

Fig. 15. Sonogram of the right parotid (P) in a patient with a history of previous melanoma excision from the right pinna. Note the intraparotid lymph node (*large arrow*) with a hypoechoic nodule in its upper pole (*small arrows*). Biopsy confirmed metastatic melanoma.

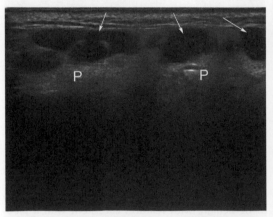

Fig. 16. Sonogram of the right parotid (P) in a patient with known Sjögren syndrome. Ultrasound shows multiple hypoechoic nodules within the superficial lobe (*arrows*). Biopsy confirmed a MALT lymphoma.

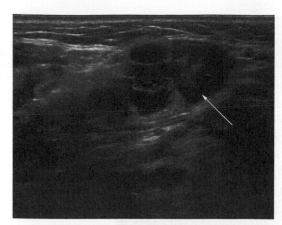

Fig. 17. MALT lymphoma infiltration in the right submandibular gland (*arrow*), in the same patient as in **Fig. 16.**

PITFALLS

Ultrasound is able to determine whether a lesion is malignant with a high sensitivity and specificity of approximately 90%.[9] However, as discussed earlier, there is overlap in characteristics of malignant and benign tumors and distinguishing between the various lesions based on ultrasound criteria alone is not always possible. Therefore, in most patients, ultrasound acts as a guide for further investigation, usually with biopsy in the first instance.

INTERVENTIONAL SALIVARY GLAND ULTRASOUND

Open surgical excision biopsy (SEB), as a method of obtaining a histologic sample, has long fallen

out of favor because of the risk of tumor seeding, facial nerve injury, facial scarring, and fistula formation.[70] The accuracy of frozen section diagnoses of the salivary gland is also controversial, with suboptimal accuracy rates for malignancy.[71,72]

Nonsurgical approaches to tissue diagnosis, particularly FNAC, have therefore been widely adopted. FNAC is a rapid and safe sampling technique that can readily be performed in the outpatient setting using ultrasound guidance. With a skilled operator and with on-site histopathologist backup and the latest laboratory techniques, FNAC has a high diagnostic accuracy.[73] However, these services are expensive and not widely available outside large and specialist centers. A recent meta-analysis of FNAC based on 64 studies concluded that FNAC had a sensitivity of 0.79 for a diagnosis of malignancy. In addition to the high false-negative rate for malignancy, the study also highlighted the significant heterogeneity in the performance of FNAC, making it impossible to provide a general guideline for its clinical usefulness.[74]

In general, FNAC is capable of a high specificity, in optimized circumstances, but has a lower sensitivity for the detection of malignancy, thus the false-negative plus high nondiagnostic rates of FNAC are disadvantages.[16,17,75]

USCB has recently been described in the diagnosis of parotid tumors, and is developing into an established technique.[15,76,77] Because USCB provides a larger sample, it potentially has a lower nondiagnostic rate, providing diagnostic biopsies without the need for on-site cytology. The core of tissue provided by USCB can also be used for immunohistochemical analysis, which can help

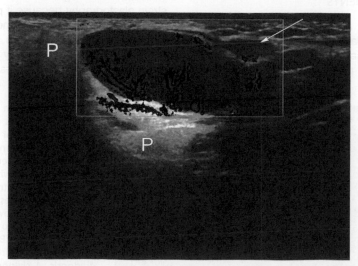

Fig. 18. Sonogram of the left parotid shows a heterogeneous, hypoechoic solid mass with chaotic internal vascularity. Biopsy confirmed infiltration with B-cell lymphoma. Note a small adjacent node (*arrow*) that appears reactive on ultrasound criteria with a large central echogenic hilum and even peripheral hypoechoic cortex.

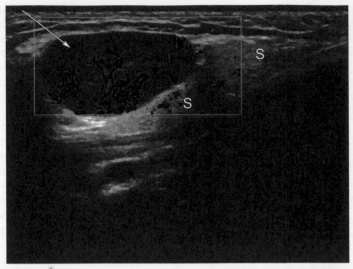

Fig. 19. Sonogram of the right submandibular space in a patient with a palpable mass. There is a mixed-echotexture mass (*arrow*) closely abutting and distorting the submandibular gland (S). Biopsy confirmed a metastasis from a squamous cell carcinoma, the lesion mimicking a submandibular lesion clinically.

with the grading and typing of parotid malignancy that is crucial in diagnosis of lymphomas. Several studies on the performance of USCB have shown the good diagnostic yields from USCB of the salivary glands.[75,78,79] A recent meta-analysis of 6 studies compiled in 2011, evaluating the accuracy of USCB in the diagnosis of salivary gland lesions, concluded that choice of the test (FNAC vs USCB) to use for an individual patient remains undefined; however, the overall accuracy of core needle biopsy is greater than FNAC in some practice settings, with less variability in performance.[80]

NEW DEVELOPMENTS

Sonoelastography is a novel imaging technique that can map the elastic properties of soft tissues.[81] A mechanical force, usually manual compression via the ultrasound probe, is applied to the region of interest. The degree and distribution of tissue deformation is detected and characterized sonographically, and is represented visually as an elastogram of the area of interest. The technique is performed using a 5-MHz to 12-MHz linear array transducer and requires a compatible ultrasound machine. Shear wave elastography (SWE) is a variation of sonoelastography.[82] In SWE, instead of the compressive force of the transducer probe the applied mechanical force consists of focused pulses of ultrasound waves termed push pulses. These induce shear waves that are detected by an ultrafast ultrasound imaging technique. This technique is thought to be more accurate than strain elastography because it produces quantitative estimates of stiffness and is less operator dependent. There have been several studies of the ability of sonoelastography to differentiate parotid neoplasms. These studies have been limited

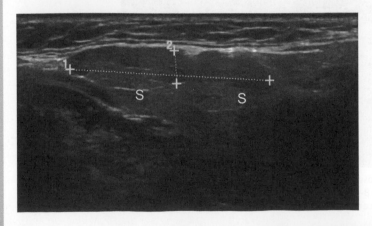

Fig. 20. Sonogram of the left submandibular gland in a patient with a hard left submandibular gland nodule. Note normal gland (S) and a geographic area of reduced echogenicity (calipers). This area is consistent with an area of chronic sialadenitis (Kuttner pseudotumor). Color Doppler assessment can help with the diagnosis, showing vessels passing from the normal to the abnormal gland with no deviation. Biopsy is not normally required to confirm this sonographic diagnosis. A sialogram may be helpful to exclude a duct stone or stricture.

by small patient cohorts and interoperator variability, and the initial results have been disappointing. Recent work focusing on identifying characteristic elastographic patterns within benign and malignant parotid lesions has shown potential in improving preoperative lesion characterization; however, biopsy is likely to remain necessary in the near future.[83,84]

WHAT THE REFERRING CLINICIAN NEEDS TO KNOW

Ultrasound is the initial imaging investigation of choice in virtually all parotid and submandibular gland masses and has a high specificity and sensitivity when differentiating benign from malignant tumors.

Ultrasound-guided biopsy of salivary lesions is a safe, rapid, and accurate method of obtaining tissue samples for analysis. Ultrasound can obviate further imaging if a lesion is sonographically confined to the superficial lobe and confirmed as benign on biopsy.

MR imaging is recommended in the imaging of deep parotid lesions or suspected malignant tumors, for which further assessment of local invasion and perineural spread is required. CT is a useful adjunct for assessing suspected bony involvement and staging lungs in malignancy.

SUMMARY

Salivary gland neoplasms constitute a wide range of benign and malignant disorders and imaging constitutes an integral part of the initial assessment of a suspected salivary gland lesion. Because of their location, the salivary glands are readily accessible with high-resolution ultrasound, which is considered the first-line imaging modality within many centers. By providing information regarding the site, nature, and extent of a disorder, ultrasound can characterize a lesion with a high degree of sensitivity and specificity. Ultrasound can also be used for image-guided intervention with FNAC or core biopsy. It provides a guide if further CT or MR imaging are required.

REFERENCES

1. Yousem DM, Kraut MA, Chalian AA. Major salivary gland imaging. Radiology 2000;216:19–29.
2. Tart RP, Kotzur IM, Mancuso AA, et al. CT and MR imaging of the buccal and buccal space masses. Radiographics 1995;15:531–50.
3. Bialek EJ, Jakubowski W, Zajkowski P, et al. US of the major salivary glands: anatomy and spatial relationships, pathologic conditions, and pitfalls. Radiographics 2006;26(3):745–63.
4. Silvers AR, Som PM. Salivary glands. Radiol Clin North Am 1998;36(5):941–66, vi.
5. Ahuja AT, Evans RM, Valantis AC. Salivary gland cancer. In: Ahuja AT, Evans RM, King AD, et al, editors. Imaging in head and neck cancer. London: Greenwich Medical Media Ltd; 2003. p. 115–41.
6. Thackray AC, Sobin LH. Histological typing of salivary gland tumors. No. 7. Geneva (Switzerland): WHO; 1972.
7. Parker GD, Harnsberger HR. Clinical radiologic issues in perineural tumor spread of malignant diseases of the extracranial head and neck. RadioGraphics 1991;11:383–99.
8. Bhattacharyya N, Fried MP. Nodal metastasis in major salivary gland cancer: predictive factors and effects on survival. Arch Otolaryngol Head Neck Surg 2002;128(8):904–8.
9. Sriskandan N, Hannah A, Howlett DC. A study to evaluate the accuracy of ultrasound in the diagnosis of parotid lumps and to review the sonographic features of parotid lesions–results in 220 patients. Clin Radiol 2010;65(5):366–72.
10. Dell'Aversana Orabona G, Bonavolontà P, Iaconetta G, et al. Surgical management of benign tumors of the parotid gland: extracapsular dissection versus superficial parotidectomy–our experience in 232 cases. J Oral Maxillofac Surg 2013; 71(2):410–3.
11. Zbären P, Vander Poorten V, Witt RL, et al. Pleomorphic adenoma of the parotid: formal parotidectomy or limited surgery? Am J Surg 2013;205(1):109–18.
12. Orloff LA, Hwang HS, Jecker P. The role of ultrasound in the diagnosis and management of salivary disease. Operat Tech Otolaryngol Head Neck Surg 2009;20(2):136–44.
13. Lee YY, Wong KT, King AD, et al. Imaging of salivary gland tumors. Eur J Radiol 2008;66(3): 419–36.
14. Bradley MJ, Ahuja A, Metrewei C. Sonographic evaluation of the parotid ducts: its use in tumor localization. Br J Radiol 1991;64(768):1092–5.
15. Howlett DC, Menezes LJ, Lewis K, et al. Sonographically guided core biopsy of a parotid mass. AJR Am J Roentgenol 2007;188(1):223–7.
16. Das DK, Petkar MA, Al-Mane NM, et al. Role of fine needle aspiration cytology in the diagnosis of swellings in the salivary gland regions: a study of 712 cases. Med Princ Pract 2004;13(2):95–106.
17. Salgarelli AC, Capparè P, Bellini P, et al. Usefulness of fine-needle aspiration in parotid diagnostics. Oral Maxillofac Surg 2009;13(4):185–90.
18. Gritzmann N, Rettenbacher T, Hollerweger A, et al. Sonography of the salivary glands. Eur Radiol 2003;13(5):964–75.
19. Koischwitz D, Gritzmann N. Ultrasound of the neck. Radiol Clin North Am 2000;38(5):1029–45.

20. Kotecha S, Bhatia P, Rout PG. Diagnostic ultrasound in the head and neck region. Dent Update 2008;35(8):529–30, 533–4.

21. Bradley MJ, Durham LH, Lancer JM. The role of colour flow Doppler in the investigation of the salivary gland tumor. Clin Radiol 2000;55(10):759–62.

22. Auclair PL, Ellis GL, Gnepp DR, et al. Salivary gland neoplasms. General considerations. In: Ellis G, Auclair P, Gnepp D, editors. Surgical pathology of the salivary glands. Philadelphia: WB Saunders; 1991. p. 312–5.

23. WHO. International statistical classification of diseases and related health problems, tenth revision, vol. 1. Geneva (Switzerland): World Health Organization; 1992.

24. Eveson JW, Cawson RA. Salivary gland tumors. A review of 2410 cases with particular reference to histological types, site, age and sex distribution. J Pathol 1985;146:51–8.

25. Spiro RH. Salivary neoplasms: overview of a 35-year experience with 2,807 patients. Head Neck Surg 1986;8:177–84.

26. Pinkston JA, Cole P. Incidence rates of salivary gland tumors: results from a population-based study. Otolaryngol Head Neck Surg 1999;120(6):834–40.

27. Kane WJ, McCaffrey TV, Olsen KD, et al. Primary parotid malignancies: a clinical and pathologic review. Arch Otolaryngol Head Neck Surg 1991; 117:307–15.

28. Batsakis JG. Tumors of the head and neck: clinical and pathological considerations. Baltimore (MD): Williams &Wilkins; 1979.

29. Takeichi N, Hirose F, Yamamoto H, et al. Salivary gland tumors in atomic bomb survivors, Hiroshima, Japan. II. Pathologic study and supplementary epidemiologic observations. Cancer 1983;52:377–85.

30. Barnes L, Eveson JW, Reichart P, Sidransky D, editors. World Health Organization classification of tumours: pathology and genetics, head and neck tumours. Lyon (France): IARC Press; 2005. p. 242–3.

31. Renehan A, Gleave EN, Hancock BD, et al. Long-term follow-up of over 1000 patients with salivary gland tumors treated in a single centre. Br J Surg 1996;83:1750–4.

32. Sikorowa L, Meyza JW, Ackerman LW. Salivary gland tumors. New York: Pergamon; 1982.

33. Tanimoto H, Kumoi K, Otsuki N, et al. Multiple primary pleomorphic adenomas in a single parotid gland: report of a new case. Ear Nose Throat J 2002;81(5):341–5.

34. Białek EJ, Jakubowski W, Karpińska G. Role of ultrasonography in diagnosis and differentiation of pleomorphic adenomas: work in progress. Arch Otolaryngol Head Neck Surg 2003;129(9):929–33.

35. Zajkowski P, Jakubowski W, Białek EJ, et al. Pleomorphic adenoma and adenolymphoma in ultrasonography. Eur J Ultrasound 2000;12:23–9.

36. Shimizu M, Ussmüller J, Hartwein J, et al. Statistical study for sonographic differential diagnosis of tumorous lesions in the parotid gland. Oral Surg Oral Med Oral Pathol Oral Radiol Endod 1999;88: 226–33, 74.

37. McGrath MH. Malignant transformation in concurrent benign mixed tumors of the parotid and submaxillary glands. Plast Reconstr Surg 1980;65:676.

38. Bryan RN, Mawad ME, Sandlin ME, et al. CT imaging of the salivary glands. Semin Ultrasound CT MR 1986;7:154–65.

39. Pollei SR, Harnsberger HR. The radiologic evaluation of the parotid space. Semin Ultrasound CT MR 1990;11:486–503.

40. Yoo GH, Eisele DW, Askin FB, et al. Warthin's tumor: a 40-year experience at the Johns Hopkins Hospital. Laryngoscope 1994;104:799–803.

41. Som PM, Brandwein MS. Salivary glands: anatomy and pathology. In: Som PM, Curtin DC, editors. Head and neck imaging. 4th edition. St Louis (MO): Mosby; 2003. p. 2005–133, 2.

42. Soler R, Bargiela A, Requejo I, et al. Pictorial review: MR imaging of parotid tumors. Clin Radiol 1997;52(4):269–75.

43. Minami M, Tanioka H, Oyama K, et al. Warthin tumor of the parotid gland: MR-pathologic correlation. AJNR Am J Neuroradiol 1993;14(1):209–14.

44. Canbay AE, Knorz S, Heimann KD, et al. Sonography and scintigraphy in the diagnosis of cystadenolymphomas (Warthin tumor). Laryngorhinootologie 2002;81:815–9 [in German].

45. Brandwein MS, Huvos AG. Oncocytic tumors of major salivary glands. A study of 68 cases with follow-up of 44 patients. Am J Surg Pathol 1991;15(6):514–28.

46. Ellis GL, Auclair PL. Tumours of the salivary glands. 3rd edition. Washington, DC: Armed Forces Institute of Pathology; 1996.

47. Seifert G, Miehlke A, Haubrich J, et al. Diseases of the salivary glands: pathology, diagnosis, treatment, facial nerve surgery. Stuttgart (Germany): Thieme Publishing Group; 1986.

48. Ethunandan M, Vura G, Umar T, et al. Lipomatous lesions of the parotid gland. J Oral Maxillofac Surg 2006;64(11):1583–6.

49. Chikui T, Yonetsu K, Yoshiura K, et al. Imaging findings of lipomas in the orofacial region with CT, US, and MRI. Oral Surg Oral Med Oral Pathol Oral Radiol Endod 1997;84(1):88–95.

50. Yoshihara T, Suzuki S, Nagao K. Mucoepidermoid carcinoma arising in the accessory parotid gland. Int J Pediatr Otorhinolaryngol 1999;48:47–52.

51. Sigal R, Monnet O, de Baere T, et al. Adenoid cystic carcinoma of the head and neck: evaluation with MR imaging and clinical-pathologic correlation in 27 patients. Radiology 1992;184:95–101.

52. Conley J, Arena S. Parotid gland as a focus of metastasis. Arch Surg 1963;87:757–64.

53. Markowski J, Gierek T, Zielińska-Pajak E, et al. Distant metastases to the parotid gland – review of the literature and report of own two cases. Otolaryngol Pol 2005;59(4):547–52.

54. Mrena R, Leivo I, Passador-Santos F, et al. Histopathological findings in parotid gland metastases from renal cell carcinoma. Eur Arch Otorhinolaryngol 2008;265(9):1005–9.

55. Howlett DC. High resolution ultrasound assessment of the parotid gland. Br J Radiol 2003;76(904):271–7.

56. Gleeson MJ, Bennett MH, Cawson RA. Lymphomas of salivary glands. Cancer 1986;58:699–704.

57. Freeman C, Berg JW, Cutler SJ. Occurrence and prognosis of extranodal lymphomas. Cancer 1972;29:252–60.

58. Zulman J, Jaffe R, Talal N. Evidence that the malignant lymphoma of Sjogren's syndrome is a monoclonal B-cell neoplasm. N Engl J Med 1978;299:1215–20.

59. McCurley TL, Collins RD, Ball E, et al. Nodal and extranodal lymphoproliferative disorders in Sjogren's syndrome: a clinical and immunopathologic study. Hum Pathol 1990;21:482–92.

60. Chiou HJ, Chou YH, Chiou SY, et al. High-resolution ultrasonography of primary peripheral soft tissue lymphoma. J Ultrasound Med 2005;24:77–86.

61. Lewis K, Vandervelde C, Grace R, et al. Salivary gland mucosa-associated lymphoid tissue lymphoma in 2 patients with Sjögren's syndrome: clinical and sonographic features with pathological correlation. J Clin Ultrasound 2007;35(2):97–101.

62. Li Volsi VA, Perzin KH. Malignant mixed tumors arising in salivary glands. Cancer 1977;39:2209.

63. Antony J, Gopalan V, Smith RA, et al. Carcinoma ex pleomorphic adenoma: a comprehensive review of clinical, pathological and molecular data. Head Neck Pathol 2012;6(1):1–9.

64. Gnepp DR. Malignant mixed tumors of the salivary glands: a review. Pathol Annu 1993;28(Pt 1):279–328.

65. Spiro RH, Huvos AG, Strong EW. Malignant mixed tumor of salivary origin: a clinicopathologic study of 146 cases. Cancer 1977;39(2):388–96.

66. Schick S, Steiner E, Gahleitner A, et al. Differentiation of benign and malignant tumors of the parotid gland: value of pulsed Doppler and color Doppler sonography. Eur Radiol 1998;8(8):1462–7.

67. Martinoli C, Derchi LE, Solbiati L, et al. Color Doppler sonography of salivary glands. AJR Am J Roentgenol 1994;163(4):933–41.

68. Beriat GK, Akmansu SH, Kocatürk S, et al. Chronic sclerosing sialadenitis (Küttner's tumour) of the parotid gland. Malays J Med Sci 2010;17(4):57–61.

69. Ahuja AT, Richards PS, Wong KT, et al. Kuttner tumour (chronic sclerosing sialadenitis) of the submandibular gland: sonographic appearances. Ultrasound Med Biol 2003;29(7):913–9.

70. McGuirt WF, McCabe BF. Significance of node biopsy before definitive treatment of cervical metastatic carcinoma. Laryngoscope 1978;88(4):594–7.

71. Carvalho MB, Soares JM, Rapoport A, et al. Perioperative frozen section examination in parotid gland tumors. Sao Paulo Med J 1999;117(6):233–7.

72. Badoual C, Rousseau A, Heudes D, et al. Evaluation of frozen section diagnosis in 721 parotid gland lesions. Histopathology 2006;49(5):538–40.

73. Robinson IA, Cozens NJ. Does a joint ultrasound–guided cytology clinic optimize the cytological evaluation of head and neck masses? Clin Radiol 1999;54:312–6.

74. Schmidt RL, Hall BJ, Wilson AR, et al. A systematic review and meta-analysis of the diagnostic accuracy of fine-needle aspiration cytology for parotid gland lesions. Am J Clin Pathol 2011;136(1):45–59.

75. Balakrishnan K, Castling B, McMahan J, et al. Fine needle aspiration cytology in the management of parotid mass: a two centre retrospective study. Surgeon 2005;2:67–72.

76. Wan YL, Chan SC, Chen YL, et al. Ultrasonography-guided core-needle biopsy of parotid gland masses. AJNR Am J Neuroradiol 2004;25(9):1608–12.

77. Naqvi SQ, Shaikh S, Shah SQ, et al. Ultrasound-guided core needle biopsy for salivary gland lesions. Gomal J Med Sci 2008;6.

78. Breeze J, Andi A, Williams MD, et al. The use of fine needle core biopsy under ultrasound guidance in the diagnosis of a parotid mass. Br J Oral Maxillofac Surg 2009;47(1):78–9.

79. Pfeiffer J, Ridder GJ. Diagnostic value of ultrasound-guided core needle biopsy in patients with salivary gland masses. Int J Oral Maxillofac Surg 2012;41(4):437–43.

80. Schmidt RL, Hall BJ, Layfield LJ. A systematic review and meta-analysis of the diagnostic accuracy of ultrasound-guided core needle biopsy for salivary gland lesions. Am J Clin Pathol 2011;136(4):516.

81. Lyshchik A, Higashi T, Asato R, et al. Cervical lymph node metastases: diagnosis at sonoelastography–initial experience. Radiology 2007;243:258–67.

82. Bhatia KS, Cho CC, Tong CS, et al. Shear wave elastography of focal salivary gland lesions: preliminary experience in a routine head and neck US clinic. Eur Radiol 2012;22(5):957–65.

83. Bhatia KS, Rasalkar DD, Lee YP, et al. Evaluation of real-time qualitative sonoelastography of focal lesions in the parotid and submandibular glands: applications and limitations. Eur Radiol 2010;20:1958–64.

84. Westerland O, Howlett D. Sonoelastography techniques in the evaluation and diagnosis of parotid neoplasms. Eur Radiol 2012;22(5):966–9.

Index

Note: Page numbers of article titles are in **boldface** type.

A

Ablation. See also Tumor ablation.
    ethanol, 56–57
    modalities for, 67–68
Abscess, pelvic, drainage of, 60
Acoustic radiation force imaging, for thyroid masses, 15
Adenoid cystic carcinomas, of salivary glands, 106
Adenomas, pleomorphic, of salivary glands, 103–104
Anesthesia, for prostate biopsy, 83–84
Antibiotic prophylaxis, for prostate biopsy, 82
Anticoagulant avoidance, before prostate biopsy, 83
Antitumor agent delivery, 57–58
Arrival time estimation, transient elastography based on, 6–7

B

Bile duct access, 58–59
Biliary ducts, tumors of, 36
Biopsy
    endoscopic ultrasound for, **43–52**
    prostate. See Transrectal ultrasound (TRUS)-guided biopsy.
    salivary gland neoplasms, 108–109
Bleeding
    after prostate biopsy, 90
    in endoscopic ultrasound, 51
Bowel cleansing, for prostate biopsy, 82–83
Brachytherapy, endoscopic ultrasound for, 54–55
Breast tumors, elastography for, 3–4, 7–8

C

Calcifications, in thyroid masses, 18
Carcinoma ex pleomorphic adenomas, of salivary glands, 107
Carcinosarcomas, of salivary glands, 107
Celiac plexus neurolysis or block, 53–54
Chemotherapeutic agents, delivery of, 57–58
Cholangiocarcinoma, 32, 34
Choledochoduodenostomy, 59
Ciprofloxacin prophylaxis, for prostate biopsy, 82
Color Doppler studies
    for prostate cancer, 84, 87
    for salivary gland neoplasms, 107–108
Compressibility relation, in elastography, 2
Computed tomography
    for cholangiocarcinoma, 32

for esophageal cancer, 44–45
for hepatocellular carcinoma, 29
for liver masses, 48
for liver metastasis, 33
for pancreatic cancer, 46–47
for salivary gland neoplasms, 102, 104, 106, 111
for tumor ablation, 71–72, 74
Contrast-enhanced ultrasound
    advantages of, 37
    contributions of, **25–41**
    disadvantages of, 37–38
    for angiogenesis monitoring, 36–37
    for biliary cancer, 36
    for gallbladder cancer, 36
    for kidney cancer, 34–35
    for liver cancer, 29–34
    for pancreatic cancer, 35
    for prostate biopsy, 87–88
    for tumor ablation, 73
    procedure for, 26–27
Cryoablation
    for kidney tumors, 71
    imaging for, 72
    patient selection for, 68–69
    principles of, 68
    procedure for, 73, 75–77
Cystadenolymphoma (Warthin tumor), 104
Cysts, ethanol ablation of, 56–57
Cytoimplant, for pancreatic cancer, 57–58

D

Deformation, of tissue, 8
Dendritic cells, for pancreatic cancer, 57
Digital rectal examination, for prostate cancer, 81–82
Direct-inversion scheme, in elastography, 7–8

E

Elastography, **1–11**
    approaches to, 1–7
    for prostate biopsy, 88
    for salivary gland neoplasms, 110–111
    for thyroid masses, **13–24**
    future of, 7–8
    harmonic, 2, 5
    nonlinearity in, 8
    physics of, 1–3
    quasistatic, 3–5

http://dx.doi.org/10.1016/S1556-858X(13)00128-X
1556-858X/14/$ – see front matter © 2014 Elsevier Inc. All rights reserved.

Moving?

Make sure your subscription moves with you!

To notify us of your new address, find your **Clinics Account Number** (located on your mailing label above your name), and contact customer service at:

Email: journalscustomerservice-usa@elsevier.com

800-654-2452 (subscribers in the U.S. & Canada)
314-447-8871 (subscribers outside of the U.S. & Canada)

Fax number: 314-447-8029

Elsevier Health Sciences Division
Subscription Customer Service
3251 Riverport Lane
Maryland Heights, MO 63043

*To ensure uninterrupted delivery of your subscription, please notify us at least 4 weeks in advance of move.

ELSEVIER

Moving?

Make sure your subscription moves with you!

To notify us of your new address, find your Clinics Account Number (located on your mailing label above your name), and contact customer service at:

Email: journalscustomerservice-usa@elsevier.com

800-654-2452 (subscribers in the U.S. & Canada)
314-447-8871 (subscribers outside of the U.S. & Canada)

Fax number: 314-447-8029

Elsevier Health Sciences Division
Subscription Customer Service
3251 Riverport Lane
Maryland Heights, MO 63043

*To ensure uninterrupted delivery of your subscription, please notify us at least 4 weeks in advance of move.

Printed and bound by CPI Group (UK) Ltd, Croydon, CR0 4YY

03/10/2024

01040378-0011